THE 1849 CHOLERA OUTBREAK IN JEFFERSON CITY

THE 1849 CHOLERA OUTBREAK IN JEFFERSON CITY

GARY ELLIOTT

THE History PRESS

Published by The History Press
Charleston, SC
www.historypress.com

Front cover: Library of Congress Prints and Photographs Division.
Back cover: Lula F. Shelton Postcard Collection, the State Historical Society of Missouri; *inset*: Wellcome Library.

First published 2021

Manufactured in the United States

ISBN 9781467148054

Library of Congress Control Number: 2020944169

CONTENTS

INTRODUCTION

History is replete with stories of multiple disasters, both natural and artificial, that have not only brought death to the masses but also, many times, created panic and distrust among the public in general. On January 24, 1848, gold flakes were discovered by James Wilson Marshall at "Sutter's Mill" in the American River near the base of the Sierra Nevada Mountains. This resulting "rush," comprising mostly men eager to travel to California seeking gold, reached its heyday in 1849. By year's end, the population of California was estimated to have increased by approximately eighty thousand over the total at the end of the previous year. Some three hundred thousand migrants came not only from the eastern and southern states but also from Latin America, Europe and even Australia. These forty-niners, as they were called, traveled any way that they could.

St. Louis, Missouri, quickly became a major travel hub for those traveling west overland. Due to its central location and large population, it became the last major port for the purchase of goods needed for the long journey. It was the "gateway to the west." This rush for gold was relatively short-lived; by 1855, it reached its end.

This rush for gold paralleled another great migration already in progress: the continuing movement of members of the Church of Jesus Christ of Latter-day Saints from various parts of the country, and Europe, to the Salt Lake Valley. Even though some of the forty-niners followed much the same path the Latter-day Saints were traveling, many of them traveled together only from St. Louis, up the Missouri River, until they parted at such cities

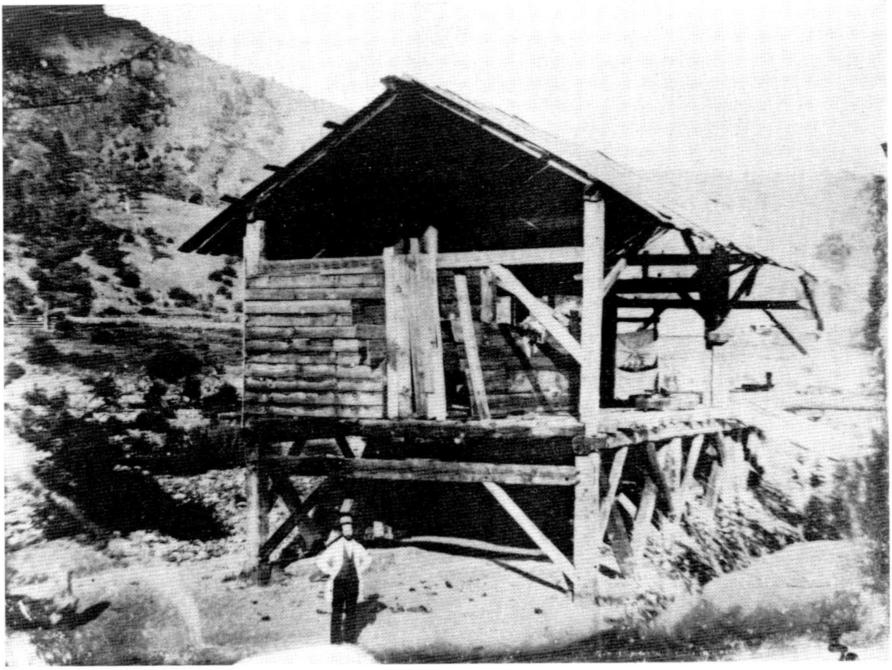

Photomechanical reproduction of an 1850(?) daguerreotype by R.H. Vance shows James Marshall standing in front of Sutter's sawmill, Coloma, California, where he discovered gold. Printed 1948. *Public Domain per Library of Congress Prints and Photographs Division.*

as St. Joseph, Independence and Westport, Missouri. Some even traveled the same route to Council Bluffs, Iowa, and on to the Salt Lake Valley. As St. Louis quickly became a gathering place for immigrants of the Church traveling to the Salt Lake Valley, William Clayton, in 1848, wrote *The Latter-Day Saints' Emigrants' Guide* to help those journeying west.

> *Guidebooks told the immigrants what supplies they needed to bring in order to survive the months-long journey with few chances to resupply, what types of draft animals to buy, the locations of the best places to camp, and where dangerous places or routes existed. Clayton's guide was so popular that non-Mormon immigrants also began to use it, and other publishers plagiarized it.*[1]

The Missouri River became the preferred route for anyone traveling to the western edges of this country. Unfortunately, river travel was not without its dangers. Steamships regularly sank or exploded on the journey from St. Louis to St. Joseph and beyond. One of the worst steamship explosions happened to the side-wheeler steamboat *Saluda*, the last hope for Mormons to make a quick departure to Council Bluffs, where they would catch a wagon train to Salt Lake Valley. On the morning of April 9, 1852, as the *Saluda* left Lexington, Missouri, its boilers exploded, disintegrating over half of the steamer.

The sound of the explosion was so loud that it was heard two miles away. Bodies, baggage and steamer parts were seen flying in all directions. Even the six-hundred-pound safe, along with the ship's bell, landed high up on the bank. Those passengers in the lower, or forepart, of the steamer were the ones who died. Those on the deck, or the stern, were numbered among the survivors. At least 28 members of the Church of Jesus Christ of Latter-day Saints lost their lives; at least as many were severely injured (there was no exact count of passengers on the boat). In addition to the members of the Church, who made up only about half of the passengers, an additional 47 passengers, along with most of the crew, perished in the\ explosion. Some reports indicated that upward of 135 persons lost their lives.

Luckily, the survivors found refuge and support from the citizens of Lexington. Not only were the travelers nursed back to health, but the locals

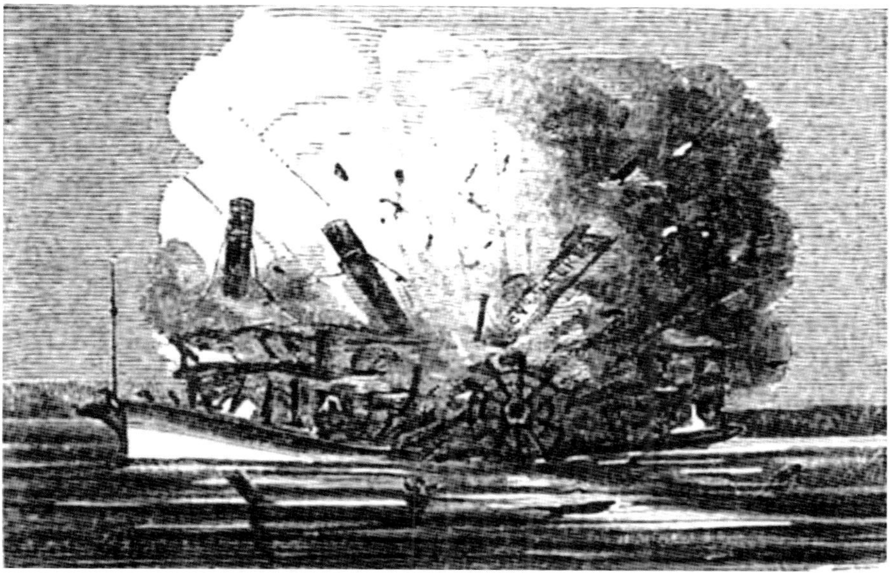

Steamboat *Saluda* river explosion, March 1852. *Westerntrips.blogspot.com*.

also raised money for those who were left with nothing and helped find homes for the orphaned children.

It was this Missouri River, and these journeys, that brought a group of forty-niners and a group of members of the Church of Jesus Christ together in a most unfortunate situation. The deaths attributed to the sideboard steamship *James Monroe* tend to get overlooked in the discussion of steamship disasters, perhaps because the deaths were not attributed to a ship's sinking or exploding, but to a cholera epidemic. Nonetheless, the loss of life was tremendous and is worthy of remembrance.

The story of the *James Monroe* was widely publicized in the newspapers of the day, with accounts appearing from New Orleans to Boston and in many large and small towns in between. This is a difficult story to accurately tell. Newspapers disagreed with each other, memories faded in later years, name spellings vary and even dates and places are sometimes incorrect. I am hopeful that I can accurately reconstruct the story of the cholera that afflicted so many individuals and families as they passed through the Jefferson City, Missouri area on that fateful day in May 1849.

The names of those who died and those who survived come from multiple sources. Some of the information about who they were has not been found; for others, I have tried my best to piece together their lives in an attempt to bring life to as many as I could. My apologies for what appears to be incorrect English usage or spellings, especially in some of the direct quotes. I have attempted to maintain the original text exactly as it was written.

E.S. Dils, one of the cholera survivors, put it best when he said, "I think the horror of the Monroe has no parallel in the history of this country; perhaps not anywhere else."[2]

1
THE PHILADELPHIA COMPANY OF LATTER-DAY SAINTS

On January 24, 1847, William Ivins Appleby of Recklesstown, New Jersey, was appointed "presiding elder in the eastern United States"[3] for the Church of Jesus Christ of Latter-day Saints. Already familiar with many of the Church members in the New England area, Appleby was constantly traveling to visit the various congregations, meeting with members and delivering sermons.

On March 17, 1849,[4] he was "called" to the church in Philadelphia, where he was asked to arrange his affairs so that he and his family could gather with other families and individuals from the Philadelphia and New England areas to begin the long journey to the Salt Lake Valley. On April 7, William Appleby and his family left Recklesstown and traveled on the Delaware River by steamboat bound for Philadelphia, where Appleby was chosen as the president of the company of Latter-day Saints, with Elders Crump and William A. Adams as counselors.[5]

Traveling the rivers to the West was not new to Appleby. He had made several trips to Council Bluffs, Iowa, so he was familiar with places like St. Louis and St. Joseph.

Appleby does not mention the first name of Elder Crump in his journal, but in an issue of *Mormon Historical Studies*, in an article by Maurine Carr Ward, "Philadelphia Pennsylvania Branch Membership: 1840–1854," a Henry Crump is mentioned. In August 1848, Appleby mentions in his journal the seventeen-year-old daughter of Brother Crump. She would have been the same age as Rebecca Franklin Crump, Henry's daughter. In 1849,

Rebecca Franklin Crump Brooks was living in St. Louis. Henry likely left the company at St. Louis to spend time with his daughter. Unfortunately, Rebecca died on July 10 of the cholera. Whether or not he was there for her death, I do not know.

The next appearance I find of him is in 1850, when he is living with his wife and son in Philadelphia. Therefore, I believe that, after visiting with his daughter, he returned to be with his family in Philadelphia. This may have been his plan from the beginning. Unfortunately, Henry never made it to the Salt Lake Valley, as he died in Maryland in 1857. Several years after his death, his wife and son were able to accomplish that migration he so desired. Henry had been a jeweler by trade.

On April 12, the company left Philadelphia bound for Pittsburgh, Pennsylvania. The company included seventy-nine individuals, men, women and children, five of whom were not members of the Church. This is a significant number of members, as the Church population in Philadelphia was around two hundred. In a letter written on August 23, 1849, Wilford Woodruff, an apostle for the Church of Jesus Christ of Latter-day Saints, stated that there were eighty individuals in the company, but only fifty of them were from Philadelphia. At least one family was from Lancaster, Pennsylvania, and several others had lived in Boston, Massachusetts, or in other New England states. Elder Woodruff was in Philadelphia assisting Brother Appleby with the preparations for their journey.[6]

The company brought with them about seventeen thousand pounds of freight. Travel arrangements were made with Captain Andrew Getty by way of the Columbia-Philadelphia Railroad for $5.50 for each full-paying passenger, half price for anyone younger than twelve and free passage for those under the age of six. It also cost $1.00 per one hundred pounds of freight. The railroad depot was located at Broad and Vine Streets. The railroad took them as far as Columbia, Pennsylvania, about 80 miles away, where they then continued by boat on the Eastern Division Canal and the Juniata Division Canal. On April 17, they arrived safe and healthy at Hollidaysburg, about 254 miles west of Philadelphia. This was at the base of the Allegheny Mountains. There, their journey changed to passage on trucks over the mountains, where they once again turned to the railroad, boarding the Allegheny Portage Railroad to convey them through the tunnels in the mountains, one of the tunnels being about five hundred yards in length.

A truck was "a small wheel; hence trucks, a low carriage for carrying goods, stone, etc. Indeed this kind of carriage is often called a *truck* in the singular."[7] Trucks were typically pulled by two horses.

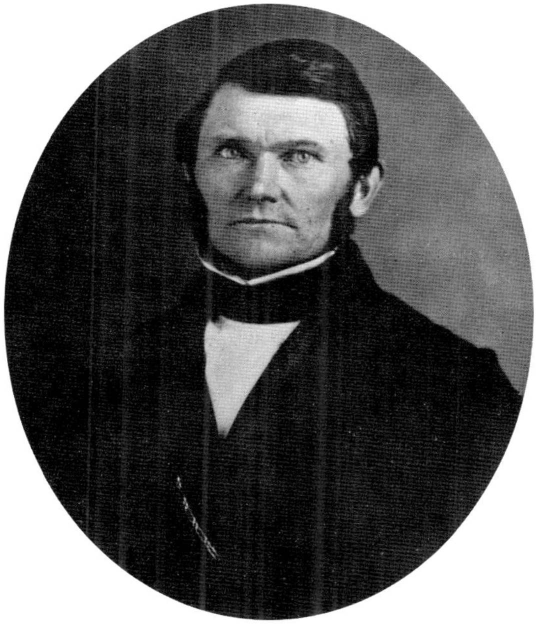

Right: Photographic copy of a daguerreotype of Wilford Woodruff, 1840–49. *Church History Library*.

Below: Early canal boats and car, Pennsylvania Railroad. *ExplorePAHistory.com*.

EARLY CANAL BOATS AND CAR; PENNSYLVANIA RAILROAD.

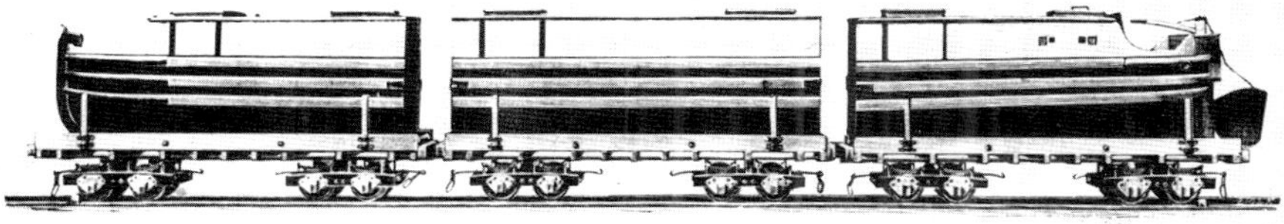

Fig. 1. SECTIONAL FREIGHT BOAT AND CARS, 1843; PORTAGE RAILROAD.

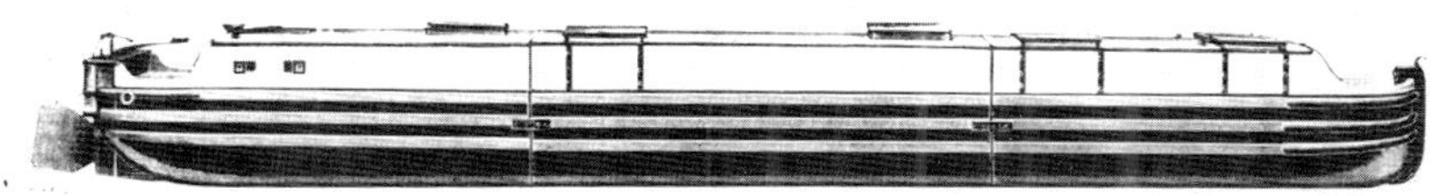

Fig. 2. SECTIONAL FREIGHT BOAT, 1843; PORTAGE RAILROAD.

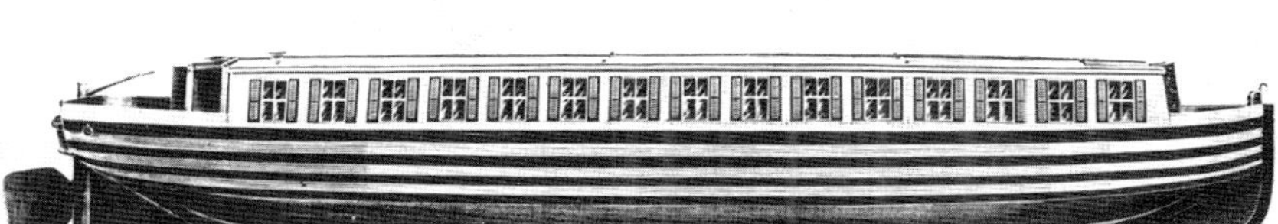

Fig. 3. PASSENGER CANAL BOAT, 1835; PENNSYLVANIA CANAL.

As the company traveled, they were known to spend much time in singing, praying and exhortation. William Appleby was regularly asked to address the Church members on different points of doctrine. On one leg of the journey, the captain became quite interested in their message and offered to arrange a meeting at their next stop, where they could preach to the locals. This they were able to do, on the deck of another steamer, with around one hundred individuals present. Several missionary tracts were given out, along with a copy of the *Proclamation of the Twelve Apostles of The Church to All Nations*. This sixteen-page proclamation, printed on April 6, 1845, was addressed:

> *To all the Kings of the World;*
> *To the President of the United States of America;*
> *To the Governors of the several States;*
> *And to the Rulers and People of all Nations:*[8]
>
> *This document was an announcement that God had spoken from the heavens and had restored the gospel of Jesus Christ to the earth. It spoke of blessings and of punishments to come, issued a warning voice, and invited all who were interested to assist in the building of the kingdom of God on the earth in preparation for the Savior's second coming.*[9]

At Johnstown, some thirty-six miles west of Hollidaysburg, they again met up with a canal boat, by which they would have traveled on the Western Division Canal. Arrival in Pittsburgh was on April 24. They gained passage on the steamer *Nominee* to carry them down the Ohio River to St. Louis.

The *Nominee* was a 212-ton side-wheel packet whose hull was constructed at Shousetown, Pennsylvania, with the steamer being completed at Pittsburgh. Its maiden voyage was in August 1848 and its first captain was Captain Joseph Smith (no known relation to the Prophet Joseph Smith). It was originally built to travel from Pittsburgh to Cincinnati but only did so during the 1849 season, after which it was sold to travel the Upper Mississippi.

On October 5, 1854, the *Nominee* had an unfortunate accident when it hit a snag about sixteen miles south of LaCrosse, Wisconsin. With a hole torn in its side, it sank in about eighteen feet of water. The steamer was a total loss. Fortunately, there was only one death. This is just one of the many ships the Philadelphia company encountered on its journey that met with a fatal ending. This was another vivid reminder of the dangers of traveling on the rivers.

The Church members had chartered exclusive rights on the steamer's deck of the *Nominee*. Several members of the company secured passage in

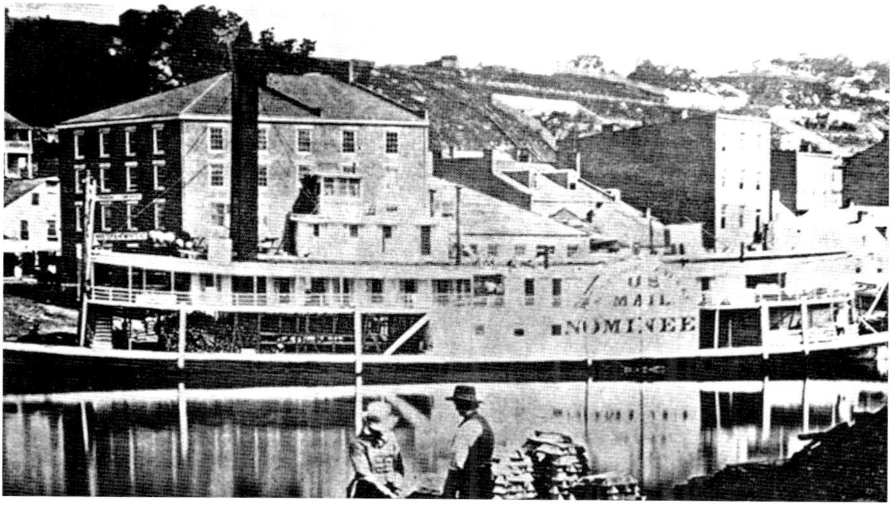

Photo of the steamer *Nominee*. *Ron Blackwell.*

cabins for the cost of eight dollars each. It also cost forty cents per hundred pounds for their freight. Because deck passage was cheaper, it provided the passenger with little else. They were not allowed in the staterooms and had to either pay for or bring their own food aboard. They were also responsible for their personal bedding. Unfortunately, sleeping on the deck provided little privacy or shelter from the noise and weather. According to federal statute, "a minimum of fifteen square feet of deck space was allotted to each deck passenger." Their space had to be "clear of obstruction, and easy of access." Furthermore, the area was to be in a "suitably enclosed deck-room, which shall be properly warmed in cool weather, and properly vented at all times."[10]

After leaving Pittsburgh on April 25, they traveled on the Ohio River bound for Wheeling, Virginia (now West Virginia), about 100 miles, arriving on the twenty-sixth. It was on April 27 that knowledge of the cholera raging on board some of the steamers up and down the rivers from New Orleans first became known to the company. Their next stop was at Cincinnati, Ohio, on the twenty-eighth, then on to Louisville, Kentucky (140 miles away), on the twenty-ninth.

On the evening of April 29, Elijah Malin (who had joined the company at Pittsburgh) became the first of the company to be seized with the cholera. Elijah was no stranger to Appleby, for they had known each other for several years. When his illness was discovered, William Appleby and Brother Crump

> *anointed, and administered to him, in the name of the Lord. He immediately began vomiting, and purging, attended with violent crampings. It appeared as though the Destroyer laid hold of us also in administering to him, for in a very short time in attending to him I became so weak and feeble I had to lie down, and Br. Crump also; while brs. Adams, Lamb, Smith, Franklin &c. attended, and incessantly administered to him, the whole long night the crampings, vomiting &c. continueing* [sic], *and such a night—such a time, and such a scene. I hope never to be my lot to witness again if it is Heavens wile. The Captain was kind in aiding and administering any thing the Boat could supply—for a while, but he gave Br. Malin up to die about 3 O'clock the following morning, but the Saints held on to him by the prayers of faith.*
>
> *About 5 O'clock this morning he appeared as though he was dying. His eyes sunk and turned back in their sockets, his flesh wasted away from off his bones to appearance quite purple in some parts of the face, and a deathly countenance in the same, his hands shriveled up, together with the finger nails purple and cold, as also his wrists, and* [his] *pulse perceptible. However he was not ceased. Working with and administering to, rubbing his hands, wrists etc. with Brandy and salt He soon after appeared to revive a little but very weak, and debilitated indeed. We passed a day here, long to be remembered. Went up on the Deck of the Boat. The Heated Steam, from the Engine, weather quite warm. Our brother at deaths door (nearly) and several others of the Company unwell, also tended to warn us to trust in God, and pray to him for deliverance, not knowing at what moment the Destroyer might attack more of us. However we committed our care to his keeping, and got a tolerable nights rest, (as Br. Malin appeared rather better) considering our situation.*[11]

The idea of rubbing "his hands, wrists etc. with Brandy and salt" may seem a little strange, but it was one of the many treatments for cholera.

> *We find in a Scotch paper (the Glasgow Herald) a description of a peculiar method of treating cholera, adopted by the Latter Day Saints, in the cases of two young ladies attacked with the disease. The process consisted in anointing with oil, prayer, brandy, psalm-singing, flannels, exhortation and hot water. The prescription was carried into effect with great vigor and perseverance throughout an entire night; and in the morning the patients were quiet and without pain, both being dead.*[12]

I am not sure that the treatment did any good other than to help the sick die quietly, and possibly a little quicker.

On the morning of May 1, the steamer came into the Mississippi River. About 1:00 p.m., a "colored" deckhand (who had a family back in Pittsburgh) died. He lay dead in his berth (adjoining Appleby's) until around midnight, when a wooden box was ready for him. He was then "carried through our midst. (The stench was intolerable) and buried along the shore." The "colored" deckhands helped in his burial.[13]

After arriving in St. Louis, Missouri, on May 2, William Appleby took a room at Augustus Farnham's residence at No. 277 Broadway. Elijah Malin was taken to his brother Samuel Malin's home, where, on May 5,[14] he passed away from the cholera. After completing a mission for the Church of Jesus Christ in Pennsylvania, Elijah was returning home to accompany his family from St. Louis to Council Bluffs, where his parents would join them for the rest of their journey to the Salt Lake Valley.

Sadly, the company found the cholera raging with full force in St. Louis. After the experiences with the cholera over the prior several days, many in the company must have been filled with fear. Once the company was in St. Louis, clothes were washed and supplies were purchased. While there, William Appleby spent time visiting some of the steamers, looking for one to gain further passage on the Missouri River for his company. The choices were limited. At this time in history, between thirty-five and forty steamships regularly traveled the Missouri River between St. Louis and Council Bluffs. On May 8, the *Missouri Republican* of St. Louis recorded twelve steamers departing the Port of St. Louis, with sixteen arriving. There were so many steamships on the Missouri River that one could almost see two steamers in view at any given time. Only one, the *Monroe*, was listed as departing for the Missouri River. In a letter to Orson Hyde, Appleby wrote: "I was on board of his Boat [the steamer *Lightfoot*], while in St. Louis, conversing with him [Captain Brooks] in regard to passage up the river, but I did not like his appearance, although he there had a member of our Church as a mate, who as I was informed he had soliciting passengers for Council Bluffs."[15]

William Appleby also tells of visiting with a company of around two hundred immigrants from England on the steamer *Mary*. He notes that several Church members on board were already suffering from the cholera and that several had died on the trip from New Orleans. If his company had been able to gain passage on the steamer *Mary*, the situation may not have turned out any better, and they may have had to wait another day for departure. The *Mary* was known to have many members of the Church on board who died from the cholera on their journey up the Missouri River.

After a few days, all but ten or twelve of the original company secured passage on the sideboard steamer *James Monroe* to carry them on to Council Bluffs. The captain of the *Monroe* was Captain John P. Moore. Those who didn't continue with the company chose to spend a few more days in St. Louis. This may have turned out to be a wise decision, as they might have avoided the cholera completely. I have not been able to find the names of those who stayed behind. Adding to their company, Augustus Farnham, his family and several other members of the Church from St. Louis joined them. William Appleby and Augustus Farnham were not strangers to each other. The Farnhams had lived in Philadelphia before moving to St. Louis.

Cabins on the *Monroe* were twelve dollars each; deck passage was five dollars. Additionally, it cost seventy-five cents per one hundred pounds for their freight. Some of the company sought passage on the hurricane (boiler) deck, but very few secured passage in one of the cabins. This move proved to be beneficial, as only a few of the deck passengers were known to have been afflicted with the cholera.

It's possible that during the journey from Pennsylvania, some members of the company took the opportunity to help the crew in such tasks as "wooding" or "scooping." "A passenger can reduce his fare by wooding on a trip....The job of cutting and carrying wood is a hard one. It should be attempted by only those used to hard work. The crew will also need help in scooping animal manure off the deck. Most captains try to clean the deck once each day."[16]

John Martin, an English immigrant, wrote: "While going up the river [Mississippi] I helped the deck hands to get fuel to the fire. For this service I got all that I could eat, and also enough for my bed mate and family of five."[17] Usually, the deck passengers were responsible for their own food and drink. River water would have been free for their use. Unfortunately, this river water could have been one of the sources for the outbreak of the cholera not only on the *Monroe* but also on the other steamships traveling the Missouri and Mississippi Rivers at this time.

Some steamers even provided cots for the deck passengers. This was not necessarily a good thing, as most of the time they were infested with lice. Therefore, many of the passengers chose to sleep on the cargo, or directly on the deck. No wonder it was typical for the deck passengers to be the ones who became ill with diseases.

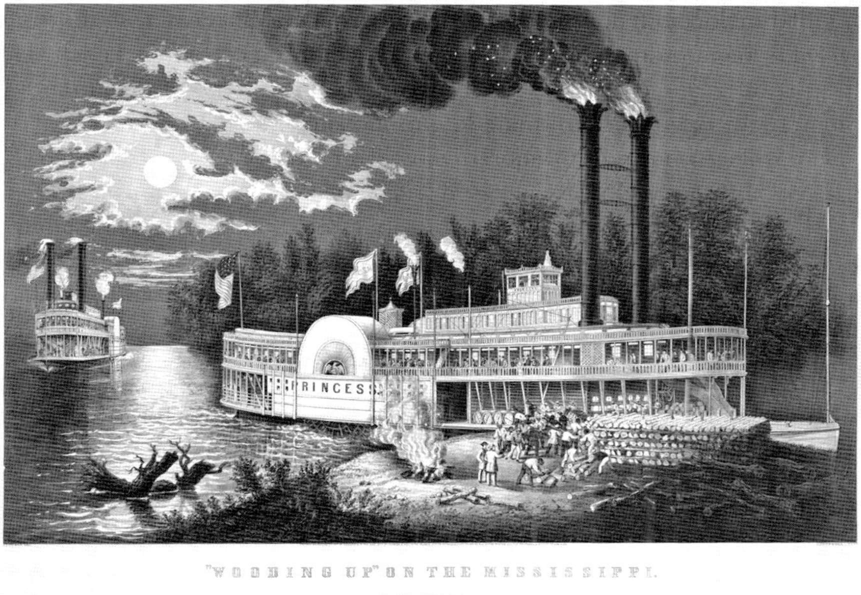

"Wooding up" on the Mississippi, lithograph by Currier & Ives, 1863. *Library of Congress Prints and Photographs Division.*

One can contrast the deplorable discomfort of those lodging on the deck with cabin passengers, many of whom came from more affluent backgrounds. They were able to enjoy "the best of everything, receiving the best food, liquor, service, comforts, and staterooms on the upper deck. In fact, the atmosphere often exceeded the best accommodations found in St. Louis hotels. Patrons walked on expensive carpets, enjoyed the view of elegant paintings, relaxed on comfortable furniture made of imported woods, in a setting embellished with an abundance of chandeliers and mirrors."[18]

There have been many conflicting reports throughout the early history of the Church of Jesus Christ of Latter-day Saints about the behavior of its members, most of which have proven to be untrue. Rice McGrew of the Jeffersonville, Indiana company recorded in his diary: "A large company of Mormons or Saints as they call themselves have embarked on our boat for Council Bluffs, some are going to remain there, others who are able are going to Salt Lake. They taken as a body are as fine intelligent looking persons as can be found, some of them are very intelligent and refined and would grace any circle of the ladies of the company in particular this is a fact."[19]

I would like to believe this behavior was the norm and not the exception.

This personal observation of Rice McGrew is in direct contrast to a letter written to the *St. Joseph's (Missouri) Gazette* by a disgruntled traveler in 1852.

> *I reached Salt Lake City too late last fall to come on, and was compelled to winter there with other emigrant's in the same fix. The treatment we received from these infernal scoundrels, is almost too bad to be believed. They shot men down in their tracks, for nothing, and confined others with a ball chain, and made them work in all weather and upon all days (for they have no Sabbaths,) and fed them only on bad bread and water; and many poor fellows suffered and died.—And what was this for? I will tell you for simply asking for the payment of what was justly due you. They would say after the work was done, that they did not owe you anything, that the people of the states treated them like dogs when they were there, and now it was their time. If the man said anything in defence and happened to say they were dishonest, and acted rascally to get their labor of a man for months and then refuse to pay, they would haul you up before a kind of court, and condemn you to from one to ten years imprisonment with a ball and chain. I have seen a man shot down at the door of their temple as he was quietly coming out of church. The cause assigned was that one of the sealed wives of the murderer had taken a fancy to the emigrant, probably not from any fault of his, for he was a married man from the Eastern States.*
>
> *It is a positive fact that a man can have as many sealed wives as he can support, and a woman can at any time be unsealed and sealed to another; in that way she may have five or six children with different fathers. When she is sealed to another, she does not take her children, but leaves them to their father; you will therefore see that in the course of 15 or 20 years, there will be hundreds of young men and girls that will not know their relationship towards each other, and inter-marriage with brother and sister to an alarming extent.*
>
> *I look upon them as the lowest people on top of the ground; the city of Salt Lake a perfect Sodom and Gomorrah, which some day if not visited by the wrath of the Almighty, I shall wonder.*[20]

What a sad tale this person told. As I look at his account more closely, I see several items that are inconsistent with official Church history and Church teachings. It is possible that either he had had a bad experience on his journey or that he was filled with hate and anger, possibly due to falsehoods he had previously been led to believe regarding those who lived in Salt Lake City.

2
THE JEFFERSONVILLE FORTY-NINERS

Around the end of January 1849, Dr. William Stephenson of Jeffersonville, Indiana, began organizing a group of men for travel to the California gold region, hence the nickname "Jeffersonville Forty-niners." Because of the expense of such a journey, Colonel Samuel H. Patterson (the prison warden) assisted in "fitting out the caravan."[21] "The prospectors had the best of everything and were well supplied with teams and mules to make the trip across the plains after the Missouri river was reached."[22]

> *Their outfit was fine. Their wagons were new, made with great care, especially for the trip. Their mules had been carefully selected, and were now quite well-broken. Their personal outfit was elegant. Their rifles—their pistols hanging in their cases—the hunting-knife thrust in the sheath, proclaimed that whatever band might attack them should count well the cost, ere it assailed that bold twenty-five* [the at least thirty-five].[23]

Around noon on May 2, Dr. Stephenson and this company of men from Jeffersonville began their journey; their eventual destination was the goldfields of California. Varying accounts put the number in this company as somewhere between twenty and thirty-five. I have been able to identify approximately thirty-five men and boys. I do not know if that is all of them, as I have found variations in spellings that could imply separate individuals, but most likely they are misspellings.

Their planned route was to travel down the Ohio River to St. Louis, where they would gain passage on a subsequent steamship and then travel the Missouri River to St. Joseph, Missouri. From St. Joseph, they intended to take the overland route by way of Santa Fe. This would not be an easy journey. Roads were rugged, and there were no luxury accommodations. "Epidemics were encountered and the plains were dotted with graves of men who had left comfortable homes and loving relatives to seek a fortune in California. Rattlesnakes and wild animals were as numerous as pebbles on the beach and these added horror to the trip."[24]

In addition to the dangers of the journey—weather and terrain, reptiles and animals, Indians and other men—many of the forty-niners also had to battle psychological stress for which they were unprepared. Many of the men had never ventured far from their homes and families for any length of time. This was especially true for the boys and younger men on this journey. Depression was real. William Swain (not of this company) recorded: "I confess that I had the blues when I found I had the prospect of being one hundred days on the plains. I had a mind to start home. But upon reflection, I think that duty to myself and *family* and relatives will not permit me to look back."[25]

As the men gathered at the dock to leave, a large crowd came to wish them a fond farewell. Included in the crowd was the superintendent of the Methodist Sabbath School. He brought a package of Bibles that his Sunday school had prepared for the forty-niners. He presented the package to them, commended them to God and went on his way. What an emotional sight this must have been. "The grief of an affectionate mother—the emotions of a sister, and the deep unutterable feelings of a confiding wife, may be imagined—not described."[26]

Having Dr. Stephenson as the leader of the company was meant to be a blessing for these men. Stephenson was a man strong in his faith. A few days before his departure, he had gone to the Methodist Episcopal Church to obtain his certificate of membership. This he placed with his most important papers so it would not be lost. For some time, he had longed to settle in California, and he saw this as the perfect opportunity to realize his dream. Before embarking on this journey, from 1845 until 1848, Dr. Stephenson had lived in the gold regions of Georgia, near the residence of his brother Matthew F. Stephenson. This event in his life likely sparked his dream of going to California. Loaded with his supply of medicine, he felt amply prepared for any medical emergencies that might confront them on their journey. Unfortunately, he was one of the first of the company to succumb to the dreaded cholera.

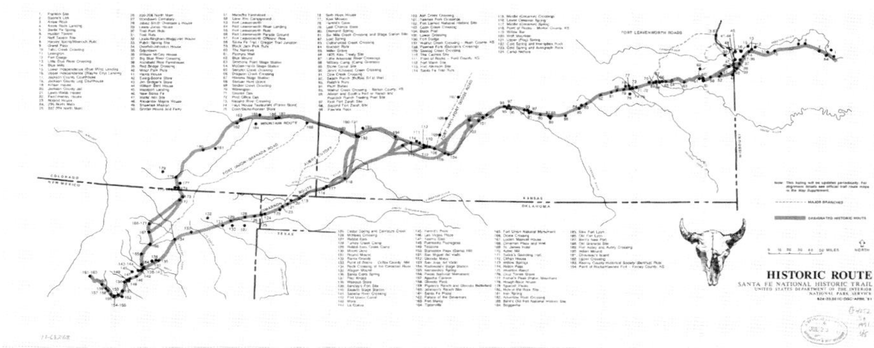

Historic route, Santa Fe National Historic Trail. *United States National Park Service. (Washington, D.C.: The Service, 1991?). Public Domain per Library of Congress Geography and Map Division.*

After leaving Jeffersonville, the company traveled the Ohio River on the steamer *North America* to St. Louis. On May 4, they reached the Mississippi River, also known as the "Father of Waters." Rice McGrew recorded in his diary his view:

> …*making our entrance of the bosom of the Father of Waters. I went on deck to have a "fair sight" of the meeting os* [sic] *waters, it was a grande sight, the expanse of the water stretching our* [sic] *before me, the low banks on one clothed with the richest verdure, on the other hand by Cairo, the town under water as some call it, but nowit(?)* [sic] *is out of the water if it has no attraction of its own, it has a part of the grand panorama that presents itself to the eye of a passerby.*[27]

The *North America* arrived in St. Louis at 10:00 a.m. on May 5. The captain of the steamer was generous enough to allow the company to leave their animals and other belongings on the boat until they were able to secure further passage on another steamer.

The *North America* was a 273-ton side-wheel packet built in Pittsburgh in 1844. It typically traveled the Ohio River between Pittsburgh and St. Louis. Unfortunately, it burned in a wharf fire at New Orleans in October 1849. It was an old boat that was docked with no cargo on board and, therefore, of little value.

Sometime on May 5, the company boarded a "lower river cotton boat," the *James Monroe*, under Captain John P. Moore bound for Independence.[28] The Jeffersonville company had with them "some forty head of horses and

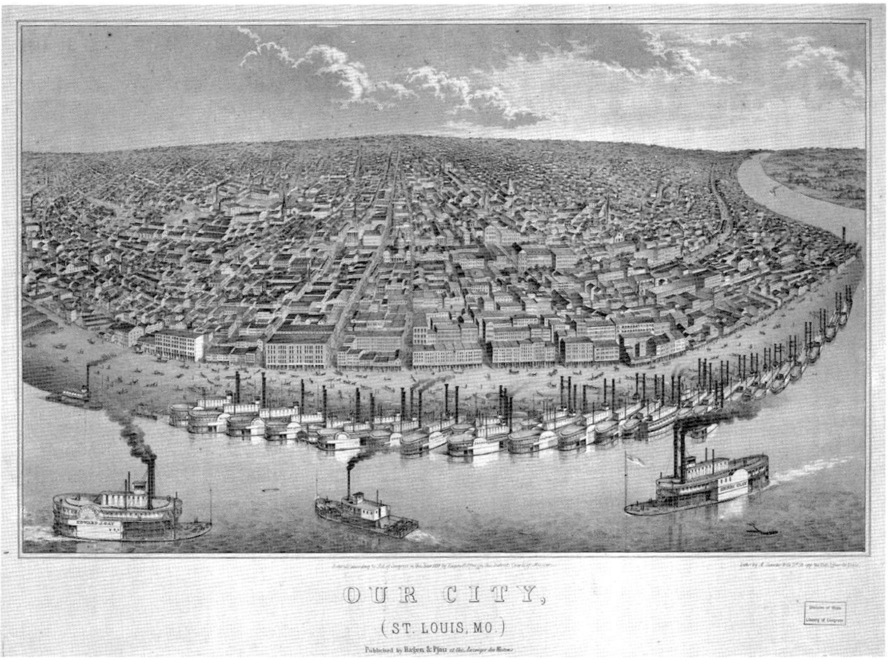

Our city, (St. Louis, Mo.). Lithograph by A. Janicke & Co., St. Louis, circa 1859. *Public domain per Library of Congress Prints and Photographs Division.*

mules, and a number of heavily laden wagons."[29] During the three days they waited on the steamer before leaving St. Louis, one member of their company succumbed to the cholera and died.[30]

For many of the company, St. Louis was the largest and busiest city most of the Jeffersonville company had ever seen. Rice McGrew, a lad of just twenty-one, wrote in his diary about what he experienced:

> *Saint Louis presents quite a handsome appearance from the river and the levee is the busiest place I ever saw, the long string of boats, high piles of every sort of Freight, immense drays and carts running up and down, draymen swearing, boatmen singing. Frenchmen jabbering, mules braying and porters and drummers for the S.Bs* [sideboards] *and Hotels worrying the life out of a man. Through such a scene I have had to force my way a dozen times today moving our waygons* [sic], *teams, etc.*[31]

The night before the steamer was to leave St. Louis (May 7), several of the company took the time to attend the theater to enjoy Dan Marble, a world-renowned Yankee comedian. "His bill announced, in big letters: 'A cure for cholera! Laugh and you will escape it.' In spite of the [cholera] epidemic the theater was crowded. The night before our departure we went on board apparently in the best of health."[32]

The sad ending to this night of enjoyment is that not only did many of the Jeffersonville company perish because of the cholera, but Dan Marble also died of the cholera at Louisville, Kentucky, on May 13.[33]

3

THE STEAMSHIP *JAMES MONROE*

The *James Monroe* was a side-wheel excursion boat with a wooden hull built in New Albany, Indiana, in 1848. It weighed 183 tons. It was 127 feet in center-line distance from the stern to the main stern transom, 25 feet wide and 5.3 feet deep from the bottom timbers to the main deck floor timbers, amidships. Its first home port was Louisville, Kentucky.[34] The steamer was believed to have been built by Isaiah King & Company of New Albany.

The sideboard *Monroe* was also described as "a vessel belonging to the southern trade, and a stranger in our river [the Missouri]."[35] Most of the excursions of the steamer *Monroe* were on the Ohio River from New Albany/Louisville to St. Louis and down the Mississippi to New Orleans. The *Monroe* was also known as a "packet." A packet was a steamship that carried both passengers and freight. The first packets began appearing on the Missouri River about 1848. Because they represented a transportation or commuter service to the public, their arrival and departure schedules were set and published in the local newspapers.

Before its voyage up the Missouri River, the *Monroe* had completed a trip from New Orleans to St. Louis, at which time it lay in port for six days while the ship "was cleaned as usual—the mattresses being sunned, the state rooms scrubbed, painted & etc. The boat then made a trip to Cairo [Illinois], took in a load of salt, and proceeded with it up the Illinois River."[36]

Presley Cordell wrote a letter to his father and said the boat "had had the cholera on her for nearly four months."[37] If Presley is correct in his observation, it may be possible that the cleaning of the *Monroe* may not have been adequate or possibly was too hurried. This could account for the fresh paint still being wet. A letter from Wilford Woodruff claims that "the cholera was on board [the steamer *Monroe*] when he [W.I. Appleby and company] went on to it."[38]

After being abandoned in Jefferson City in May, the *Monroe* was back in operation on the Missouri River by September; by November, it was running as a packet traveling from St. Martinville, Louisiana, to New Orleans with Captain W.S. Johnson in command.[39] On the morning of March 27, 1854, between 2:00 and 3:00 a.m., while traveling from New Orleans to the Yazoo River in Mississippi, the *Monroe*, loaded with dry goods and groceries, struck a log at Cowpen Point, about five miles above Natchez, Mississippi, and sank, all in less than five minutes. This was during a windstorm that had made the river rough.

Since there was only one passenger aboard, deaths were confined to the steamer's crew. The seventeen lives lost included the mate, fifteen deckhands and firemen, along with a "Negro" woman who belonged to Mr. Partee. All were drowned. The sole cabin passenger, along with the captain and clerk, were among those who survived. The twenty or so survivors were rescued hanging on to the hurricane deck as it floated away. The *Monroe* had been valued at around $75,000 with a cargo worth between $50,000 and $75,000. Even the safe, which contained $11,000 in cash, was lost. The *Monroe* was considered old, with engines that "had been used in four other boats—the Jo Davies, Col. Clay, and two Reindeers, all of which boats had sunk."[40]

Because of the dangers of river travel, and with great odds that a steamship would be involved in a boiler explosion (steamers were made primarily of wood), the average life span of a steamboat was five years. An older boat would be less reliable and would require many more repairs. Built in 1848, the *Monroe* had outlived its average life span.

It was said of its sinking that "the hull of the Monroe went down immediately, but the cabin doated off, and those who clung to it were rescued by the Southern Belle....As the steamer sunk she capsized, and the cabin separated from the hull when it was towed to the shore."[41]

4
THE MISSOURI RIVER JOURNEY AND DEATH BY THE CHOLERA

During 1849, most of the steamships that traveled on the Missouri River (and the Mississippi) carried the cholera. The steamer *Mary* is one example.

> *The steamer Mary bound for Council Bluffs with 300 passengers, mostly Welsh Mormons on the trip between St. Louis and Glasgow, had 21 cholera deaths. By the time the Mary arrived in St. Joseph, there were 47 cholera deaths which occurred during those 480 miles, averaging a little over one death every ten miles.*[42]

The interesting contrast between the steamers *Mary* and *Monroe* is that, it was reported, "the mortality [on the *Mary*] was confined solely to the Mormon emigrants on deck,"[43] while on the *Monroe*, there were very few deck casualties.

Even the steamer *Lightfoot*, on which most of the surviving members of the Philadelphia and St. Louis companies eventually continued their journey, was not exempt from the cholera. It was said that about thirty passengers died on the steamer *Mameluke* between New Orleans and St. Louis. Many of these survivors would have transferred to the *Lightfoot* at St. Louis. Unfortunately, the *Mameluke* (also spelled *Marmaduke*) was one of the steamboats that burned in the "great conflagration" that destroyed twenty-three steamships on May 17, 1849, in St. Louis.

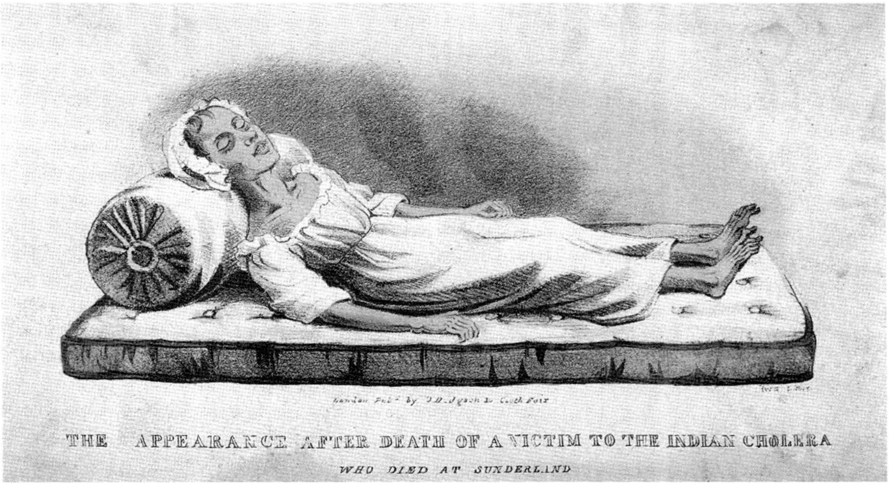

A dead victim of cholera at Sunderland in 1832. *This file is licensed under the Creative Commons Attribution 4.0 International license.*

Shortly after the *Lightfoot* departed Jefferson City, there were two more deaths among its original passengers. These victims were buried in wooden boxes along the shore. Even after the *Lightfoot* left Jefferson City, there were reports of deaths and burials near the mouth of the Grand River. There was even one false report that said "the Lightfoot was deserted and still lies up the river."[44]

William Swain wrote in his journal:

> *[Other reports told of cholera raging "with great violence raging on board several steamers, one of which…was entirely abandoned and left tied to the shore." On another, cholera broke out "with virulence" the very first night out of St. Louis: "Under the unfavorable circumstances of irregular diet and a crowded and dirty steamer, its effects were quick and deadly. A great panic ensued, and many of the noisiest braggarts became suddenly endowed with lamblike meekness. Some eighteen or twenty poor fellow died and were laid on the deck till enough corpses accumulated, when they were buried, wrapped only in their blankets, in shallow holes hastily dug by the deck hands on the river islands, the boat barely stopping long enough for the purpose."]*[45]

J.S. Holliday remarked in a footnote in the same source, "This abandoned steamer was probably the *James Monroe*."[46] Interestingly, the above quote appears to be an afterthought attached to the date of April 28, the day on which Swain arrived at Jefferson City, another demonstration of how widespread the news of the cholera in Jefferson City was.

Then there were the accounts, in later years, that appear to be describing the steamer *Monroe* but with incorrect information. One example of possibly inaccurate information is a newspaper report in 1904:

> *The saddest of all incidents that ever occurred on the Missouri was that which happened to the steamer Haidee in 1859. The boat left St. Louis, having on board a company of California emigrants, consisting, perhaps, of 200 people. At Jefferson City the cholera broke out on the boat. She was tied to the bank, the crew deserted her, and as far as the writer can recall the circumstances, not over half a dozen persons escaped the ravages of the dread disease. The emigrants buried their own dead, as far as they could, the last of them being left dead on the boat. In due time the boat was fumigated, an attempt made to again put her into commission, but without success.*[47]

Then there is the 1906 account, which states:

> *Only one season is recalled when the town* [St. Louis] *had any relief from this most terrible monotony. That was during the winter of 1848, when the steamer Haidee got caught up the river a little too late and was frozen in at the town, remaining all winter and going out with the ice in the spring. This was the same steamer upon which cholera broke out in the summer of 1850 just below Jefferson City. She was tied up to the bank, several of her officers and crew died and the remainder deserted, the passengers, possibly 200 emigrants, being left to the mercy of the disease. Not one of them was allowed to visit Jefferson City and no one from the city was allowed, had any one been willing, to go to their relief. They were closely quarantined by the farmers of the surrounding country and left to work out their own salvation. If the writer remembers correctly, only two persons of all the passengers were found alive when the disease had run its course—a mother and her boy, a lad 8 or 10 years old. The mother died soon after being taken from the boat and the boy was adopted by Mr. Emery Livermore, at one time connected with the wholesale grocery house of Livermore, Cooley & Co. which for years did business well up on North Second street, St. Louis.*[48]

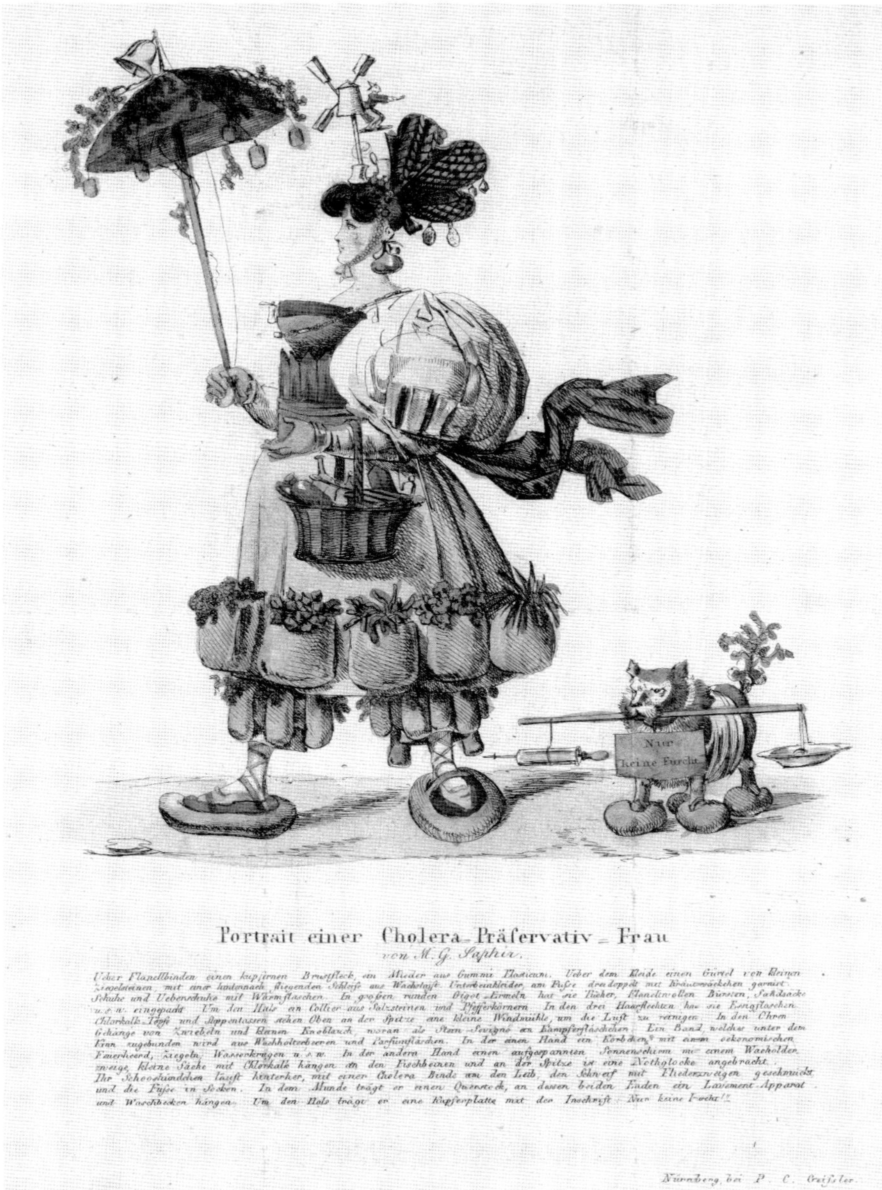

Portrait of a "cholera-preservative woman." Text below describes the clothing and devices she and her dog use to ward off the disease. Peter Carl Geissler, engraver, circa 1850. *Public domain per Library of Congress Prints and Photographs Division.*

There are just too many similarities between these two newspaper recollections with the landing of the steamer *Monroe* to not be descriptions of the same event. Unfortunately, memories faded in later years.

Of all the steamers traveling with the cholera on the Missouri River at this time, only the *Monroe* is known to have docked at Jefferson City. It was said that "every part of the boat [was] crowded to suffocation" with passengers.[49] The idea that a steamboat would be this "crowded" was not unusual. In April 1849, Lewis D. Cook wrote a letter to his mother in which he stated: "The *Amelia* was crowded from stern to stern, and so is every other boat that starts from St. Louis rendering it difficult to secure a birth [*sic*] unless you go and engage your passage a day or two before a steamer leaves, taking up your lodgings on board at the same time."[50]

There is no definitive account of how many passengers were actually on board the *Monroe*. If most of the cabins were full, with most of the Latter-day Saints having secured passage on the deck, it is possible, because of all the freight and personal belongings of the passengers, that the steamer was overcrowded. One account says there were "about one hundred fifty passengers on board the boat."[51] Still another one says, "there were over three hundred Mormon deck and at least one hundred cabin passengers, mostly bound for the Golden State, with a vast amount of goods, stock, etc."[52] This account, recollected in 1892, is inconsistent with other accounts; however, the *Monroe* likely took on board a large contingent of other passengers at St. Louis that is not mentioned anywhere else. One account even said:

> *This company of Californians which left Jeffersonville and this city some three weeks since have lost about half their number from death by the dread disease. This company embarked on board the steamer* Monroe *at St. Louis, on Sunday, the 6th inst., and were to leave for Independence Monday morning, a significant number of passengers having already taken passage. On that morning, however, a large number of Mormon passengers were received on board by the Captain.*[53]

This account tells us that the company from Indiana was not the first to board the steamer and that quite a few "Mormons" boarded after them. This would tend to confirm that there could have been more than the two companies on board. Unfortunately, I have been unable to find any additional information on who else might have been on board.

Another interesting account is given in the *Journal of Elisha Douglas Perkins*, in which he says:

> *This vessel* [the *Monroe*] *left St. Louis last week with about 100 cabin passengers & 50 deck, all well, at the mouth of the Missouri the Cabin passengers began to be attacked & before reaching Jefferson City 150 miles—70 of them died; at the city the boat was deserted & all fled for their lives. Of the 100 passengers only three are now living & well!... One company from Indiana were on board, of 27 men with their wagons, baggage &c only two of them were spared to tell the sad tale to relatives & friends.*[54]

As an estimate for the number of passengers on board, 150 is not bad. But in the next line, he refers to only 100 passengers. Another problem is when he refers to 70 passengers having died before reaching Jefferson City and then says that only 3 are living. Additionally, he refers to only 2 survivors out of 27 of those from Indiana. That is not a bad estimate, but at least 13 survivors have names, with only 2 or 3 of them continuing their journey to California. That could be where some of the confusion on the number of Indiana survivors comes from.

An additional account states: "Together with three other California expeditions, also largely composed of Indianians [*sic*], we were compelled to wait an entire week on the steamer, which was being refitted."[55] Nowhere else have I found evidence of additional companies from Indiana on board the *Monroe*, and the idea of waiting on the ship for a week is inconsistent with their arrival and departure date in St. Louis. Other accounts have told of the *Monroe* being painted and cleaned, which would accord with the refitting statement. It is also possible that the other three California expeditions referred to secured passage on another steamer. There is also this account: "In due time the James Monroe reached Jefferson City loaded to the water's edge and nearly every soul aboard of her flat of his back with cholera."[56]

It is logical to assume there were many other passengers on board the *Monroe* besides the companies from Indiana and Pennsylvania, but I find it odd that no one talks about death, or survival, among those individuals. Then there is the account that says: "Of 400 souls there was barely two scores of survivors at the end of four or five days."[57]

There is also the account written by a reporter for the *Cincinnati Commercial* who appears to have been in Jefferson City near the time of the steamer disaster. He writes that "only 23 out of 159 are left to tell the tale, and perhaps among these 23, death has already set his mark."[58]

Regarding the possible overcrowding of the *Monroe*, we have the authors' words in *The World Rushed In*:

> *[Other river steamers were equally crowded with: "a dense medley of Hoosiers, Wolverines, Buckeyes, Yankees, and Yorkers, including blacklegs, and swindlers of every grade.... The decks above and below exhibited a stupendous assortment of wagons, horses, mules, tents, bales, boxes, sacks, barrels, and camp kettles; while every cabin and stateroom was an arsenal of rifles, fowling pieces, bowie knives, hatchets, pouches powder horns, and belts." "Every berth was full, and not only every settee and table occupied at night, but the cabin floor was covered by sleeping emigrants."]*[59]

Another detailed description of the problem with overcrowding comes from the *Louisville Journal*:

> *The number of deaths on the Western steamboats is strictly regulated by the comforts and accommodations they afford passengers.—On the boats engaged in the Louisville and New Orleans trade, the deaths have been comparatively few, because their decks have not been so crowded, and are kept clean. Boats have passed here within whose narrow decks from three to five hundred human beings have been densely stowed or packed. The filth and stench on such boats are almost insupportable. The food used is one of the most unwholesome kind, and the atmosphere which is breathed is impure in the extreme. Under such circumstances, nothing but disease and death can rightfully be expected. All the laws of health are put at defiance. As well you might expect health in the Black Hole of Calcutta when crammed with human beings, as on the deck of a steamboat, where hundreds are huddled together so thick that those who are well in passing to and fro, tread upon the wretched sick who cannot get out of the way.*[60]

There is also the account from William Swain relating his experience on the *Amelia*, in which he said that it "was crowded to overflowing with 250 tons of freight and one hundred passengers."[61]

Determining the exact number of passengers aboard the *Monroe* is virtually impossible, but estimating the number is a little easier. In 1866, the crew on the *Ontario* included: "a captain, two clerks, two pilots, two engineers, two mates [boatswains], a steward, two watchmen, one head cook, two assistants, one hostellier (barkeeper), seven cabin boys, a porter or baggage man, eight deck hands (white), four firemen, nineteen negros for all the work of the boat, and one chamber-maid. Total crew—57."

Meanwhile, "the crew of the *Deer Lodge* was: 30 deckhands, handy man, all negros; 2 pilots, 2 mechanics, 2 boatswains (mate), 6 firemen, 1 clerk,

1 barkeeper, 3 or 4 cooks, 1 barber who was also the baggageman, 6 chambermaids and one laundress. All white but the barber, the chambermaids and the cook."[62]

This makes a total crew of fifty-six or fifty-seven.

I am not sure if there is much difference in crew size between a stern-wheeler and a side-wheeler, but, according to the above statements, there could have been a crew of approximately fifty-seven. Then there was the company from Indiana numbering around thirty-five and the combined companies from Philadelphia and St. Louis numbering around one hundred. There also had to have been others not of these companies on the steamer, but I have found the names of only two.

This number falls to less than 200 on board the *Monroe*. However, if one uses the equation that deck passengers usually number three or four times that of cabin passengers, and we know that most of the Indiana company was lodged in cabins (with a few of the others also being in cabins), that would bring the estimate of the number of those passengers lodging on the deck to between 105 and 140. The use of the higher number, 140, would estimate total passengers and crew to be around 232. Whether that number represents overcrowding or not would also be directly related to the size of the steamer, the number of passengers and the total amount of cargo it was carrying.

5

DEPARTURE, DEATH AND ADVENTURE AT JEFFERSON CITY

When the various parties booked passage on the *Monroe*, they did so with the expectation that the captain and his crew had a moral responsibility

> *for the comfort and health of their passengers. They know how many persons can be safely and comfortable accommodated on their boats, and when they, for the sake of a few dollars, take on board two or three times as many persons as they can accommodate, they willfully peril the health and lives of their passengers. The wretched immigrants from Europe that have recently arrived at New Orleans are anxious to reach their destination, and, knowing nothing of the capacity of a steamboat, they huddle together in great numbers, ignorant of the dangers and discomforts they thereby subject themselves to. But the officers of the steamboats know that when they suffer these poor ignorant emigrants to cram the decks of their boats, suffering, disease, and death, must afflict them from the moment when they leave port until they reach the port for which they are bound. How any man who has a heart in his bosom can consent to have his boat overcrowded at such a season as this, when he knows that the effect will make his boat a hospital where ship-fever and cholera will be a frightful execution, is more than we can conceive. It often happens that within the short period of a week, the deck passengers are decimated, and indeed it sometimes happens that the mortality is greater even than ten percent of the whole.*[63]

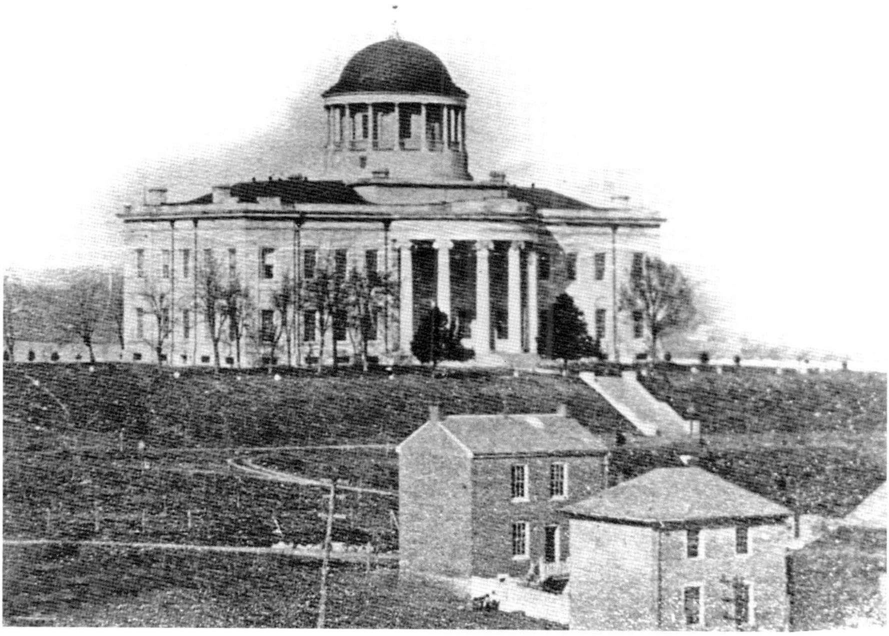

Second Missouri State Capitol Building, 1900. MS066 Peter Herman Rackers Photograph Collection. *Public domain, courtesy of Missouri State Archives.*

There are several conflicting accounts of when the cholera started on the steamer. Some say that when the company of forty-niners from Indiana boarded the steamer, the cholera had already attacked many of the Church members from Philadelphia and St. Louis. This idea is inconsistent with previous statements that the company from Indiana boarded first. Others say the cholera was already on board when those bound for the Salt Lake Valley boarded. It's all a matter of perspective, and possibly the cholera was found early on among members of both companies. But it is also possible that it hadn't fully manifested itself yet.

On May 7, before leaving St. Louis, several passengers were attacked with the cholera, possibly a deckhand and one or two of the Jeffersonville company. They were immediately removed from the boat. Preston Samuels was among those attacked and left in St. Louis with two companions from the Jeffersonville company to help care for him. "He was removed as soon as possible to the Hotel of Invalaides [*sic*], the best Physicians in the city engaged, but they gave us no hope for his recovery."[64] He soon perished with the cholera. I do not know who his companions were or what happened to them.

On the morning of May 8, around 4:00 a.m., the *Monroe* officially left St. Louis. Shortly after leaving, one of the Jeffersonville company who had gained passage in a wagon box on the hurricane (upper) deck became ill and died (on May 9). A wooden box was prepared for him, and he was buried at a "woods landing" that morning around 11:00.[65] E.S. Dils, of the Indiana company, remembered:

> *During the night some one tapped on my cabin door and called: "Get up Dills! McGlemery is dead!" I jumped into my clothing horror struck. The man had been in rugged health only an hour before, I looked at the body; it was black, shriveled and unrecognizable. Another man named Williams, from Port Fulton* [Indiana] *died shortly after. The bodies were taken ashore, and a man named Chaflin stayed with them. I believe he, too, died.*[66]

On May 8, Rice McGrew wrote in his diary regarding the death of McGlenry:

> *Got up this morning and found taht* [sic] *the man who was suffering from the Cholera had died during the night and found all our company in consternation. Edward Maglone* [McGlenry] *had been attacked during the night with that most dreadful disease the Cholera. I asked the Doctor what he thought of the case, "He will surely die" he answered. It is useless to try to describe my feelings. I went to bed the night before and left him up, apparently well as a man as there is in the company, got up in the morning, found him dying. We did all that our minds or others coucld* [sic] *suggest, but it did no good, he died in greeat* [sic] *agony and before his corpse cold, another of our company, a roommate of the deceased Mr. Preston Samuel.*[67]

It was the standard practice that, when a passenger died, the body would be placed in a crude wooden box, with the boat stopping to allow people to dig a shallow grave in which to inter the box. Unfortunately, this shallow grave remained unmarked until the river's constantly changing course invaded the sacred spot where the coffin lay. It was not unusual to see coffins sticking out of the ground or even floating down the river. The ship's carpenter had the task of constructing the coffins, possibly as soon as someone became sick, with the intent of disposing the body as quickly after death as possible.

About the time of McGlenry's burial, the ship's pilot, Joseph Ponto of St. Charles, Missouri, and one of the engineers became ill with the cholera. Both died that night. What a scene of death it must have been on the *Monroe*. E.S. Dils described the scene:

> *We were more than anxious to get away. In the morning we cast loose* [from St. Louis] *and steamed up the river for St. Joe, hoping to leave the cholera behind us, but were doomed to a terrible disappointment. After but a few hours' run a number of the Mormons died. The boat was stopped to bury them on a sandbar. It was only two hundred miles to Jefferson City, but we were two days and two nights getting there. Our boat was becoming a floating hearse, and panic held possession. It was awful; lamentations, prayer, curses, dying agony, shrieks of pain, mingled with thump, thump, thump of the engines. Then a sudden stoppage, a hastily scooped hole in the sand. Another one had been left behind.*[68]

Also, on May 9, one of the members of the Philadelphia company died after succumbing to the cholera. He lingered longer than any of the previous victims. Unfortunately, his name was not mentioned. How many nameless individuals who died is not known. Fortunately, we do have the accounts of some of those named, Dr. Stephenson being one of the first.

> *At ten o'clock, Wednesday night* [May 9], *he* [Dr. Stephenson] *stood on the guard conversing with his nephew* [E.S. Dils]*; he had just come down from the room of the dying pilot* [Joseph Ponto]. *He remarked, that it seemed singular that the disease was utterly unmanageable—that he never saw it before so fatal—but, for himself, he never felt better in his life—had no symptoms of disease. In two hours he was struggling with the angel of death! He was attacked soon after lying down. With the utmost self-possession he ordered the application of remedies: they were powerless. He saw he must die. He called for Mr. Dorrough, one of the principal men of the company—gave him some directions as to his effects and the company—then requested that all should leave him. He desired, in his little room, to meet his God in solemn communion, ere, an "undressed spirit," he stood before his bar. He suffered severely, several hours, on the boat. Thursday morning the boat reached Jefferson City. Many were sick and dying. The brave officers and crew deserted the vessel! They landed—conveyed the Doctor to a hotel, and laid him on a mattress. He suffered two hours, when the "golden bowl was broken"—the spirit was with his God!*[69]

The first impressions of seeing Jefferson City must have been exciting to the passengers, or at least to those who were able to enjoy it. Peter Decker, who traveled on the Missouri River by steamer, passed Jefferson City on April 13 and recorded in his diary this description of what he saw: "Passed Jefferson City the Capitol of Mo. Located on hill. Penitentiary in view. A fine State House of lime stone, two stones high on the side a semi-circle assent to the door supported by 5 Iconic columns."[70]

E.D. Perkins provides us with a more detailed view of the capitol.

> *Jefferson City the Capital of the great Missouri State, is built on a succession of small bluffs & has a very irregular appearance.*
>
> *The State House standing on a bold elevation about 100 feet above the river is built of the Missouri marble a cream colored stone which polishes well but seems to crumble on exposure to the air, & I noticed many of the stones in the building were broken into perhaps a dozen pieces. The State House has a semi circular portico with white marble pillars on either front & with its dome which more resembles that of the St. Charles Hotel in New Orleans than any I ever saw presents altogether a fine appearance.*[71]

My favorite view of Jefferson City comes from the writings of J. Goldsborough Bruff, who stopped here on April 20. He wrote: "We stopped a few minutes at Jefferson City; whose State House, about 3 miles above, looked like a small edition of our Capitol, at Washington. The State Prison, is a fine building also—City looks very neat—High round hills about it, while the opposite banks are low & thickly wooded."[72]

His description fits very well with the city's working hard to keep the community clean and free of diseases.

William Appleby was no stranger to Jefferson City. On November 19, 1847, he had the opportunity to stop there on his travels from Philadelphia to Council Bluffs. His account says that he:

> *Stopped there a few Hours. I took a stroll through the City to view it. It being the Capital of the State of Missouri. It is situated on rising and broken ground, with large hills—valleys and gulleys, interweaving, with houses scattered here and there, some brick, some frame, and others Logs &c The Streets are not paved, very muddy and tolerable wide. The State House is the only building of any note, that I observed in the place, that is quite a large Square building, four Stories high, built of White Limestone with a Cupola on a sort of a Tower on the top. It is situated on a hill*

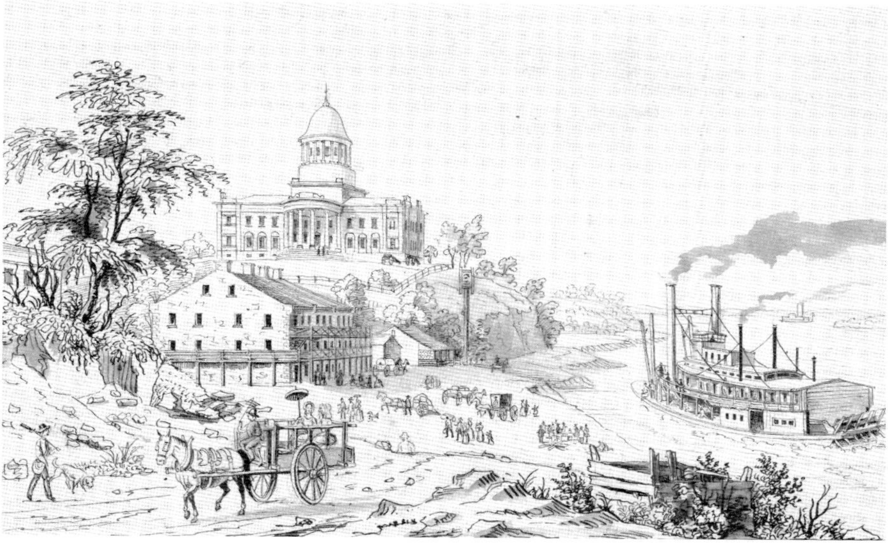

Jefferson City, Missouri, by Edward Sachse, about 1845. *Legends of America*.

> *of considerable eminence, commanding the River. I also observed one or two Churches, Two Printing Offices, two Hotels, and plenty of grocery's* [saloons], *and a State Prison. How many convicts within I do not know. Population about 12 Hundred!*[73]

As the *Monroe* approached Jefferson City, William Appleby recorded in his journal:

> *No less than four of our Company I saw lying on the floor in the Ladies Cabin dieing* [sic] *at one time, others of the Californians died while carrying them into town, from off the Boat, or soon after they had been conveyed to the Hotels, or evacuated houses in the City. The Boat being unable to proceed any further. Those that were able were advised to remove from off the Boat immediately, and endeavor to procure places for themselves, families &c. which were quite readily obtained, as a great many Houses in Jefferson City had been vacated by persons gone to California. Accordingly we obtained two or three large Houses together where the greater part of the Company of Saints, and those journeying with them, that were able, together with a great portion of their baggage were removed, some staying on board, together with some of the citizens to attend to the dying & the Californans* [sic] *going to the Hotels, chiefly.*[74]

The *Jefferson Inquirer* reported that five deaths took place on board the steamer between St. Louis and Jefferson City.[75] It was also said that thirteen of the Jeffersonville company died with the cholera before they reached Jefferson City. On May 10, Captain Val Jordon, the barkeeper, along with several of the California company, together with William Hand; William A. Adams, his wife and two of his daughters; and William Hampton's wife (all of the Philadelphia company) became ill. Except for a young daughter of William A. Adams, all died by the afternoon. On reaching Jefferson City about 10:00 a.m., the steamer had no option but to land there, as so many of the crew had died, and they didn't have enough workers left to continue their journey.

Dr. Stephenson was being carried

> *ashore on a cot, determined to go no further, and behind us came the panic-stricken mob of passengers, crew and officers, pouring ashore and the cholera came with them. It was a horrible scene. The Mormons spread out along the bank, vomiting and lying down to die by the score. The Monroe and her terrible cargo created a panic in the town. We had brought them the plague. At first they would not permit us to enter the place and we took our dying captain (Dr. Stephenson) into an empty home, where he breathed his last. Then they allowed us to go to one of the hotels, and there the boys began to die. They died like flies. Those who were able had to nurse and care for five and six sick men. But it was soon over and only seven of the thirty were left.*[76]
>
> *After the Doctor's death, the next of the company who fell, was William Edgington, a young energetic man, to whom, next to Doctor S., the company looked for counsel and direction: he left a widow and orphans. On Friday night, or Saturday morning, Wm. B.* [D.] *Beach breathed his last. He was the child of many prayers and fond hopes. He had been a student of Asbury University; but his health was gone. He went out under the care of Dr. S., hoping to find, in the change of life, diet, air, scenery, etc., a restoration to health and activity. Vain hope! he was seized—lived a few hours, and died, asking them to remember him to his parents!*
>
> *Time rolled on. Ere Sabbath dawned upon the world, John Edgington, Rice M'Grew, and William Stephenson, the son of Dr. S., were numbered with the dead! Room will not admit of a notice of these young men. They were the beloved of many hearts. Young Stephenson died in the Episcopal church—M'Grew in the Presbyterian church. Sabbath morning Mr. Davenport died.*[77]

Also numbered among the dead was William Beach, the son of William D. Beach.

Additionally, Mrs. Sabra Granger of Commerce was listed among the dead. She was with the company from St. Louis. There were also at least five females whose names were not known. Also, Lavina Hodges, the wife of John Hodges, was listed among the dead. John Hodges left the boat around 10:00 a.m. on Saturday, May 12, and records state that, up to that time, fifty-three persons had died. That number could include not only those of the Philadelphia company but also members of the ship's crew and those of the Indiana company. In addition to the passengers from the Indiana and Pennsylvania companies, there were others not of their groups onboard. It was reported that "Mr. John Hubbard, principal of the Bowling Green [Missouri] Academy, was amongst the passengers of that ill-fated boat, and has not been heard from since."[78] Unfortunately, he is only one of two, not of either company, who was named.

Along with no known list of all the passengers, it is also difficult to know how many died of the cholera. One narrative, provided by E.S. Dils in 1904, said: "every other who started from Clark county [except for E.S. Dils and Henry Dellinger] being cut down by the scourge of cholera before they were much more than started….The majority of those who were on that ill-fated vessel hailed from this county and its sister, Floyd."[79]

There are several problems with this memory. Dils says that only two survived (not including himself). This is inconsistent with other accounts and with the list of survivors provided later in this book. Possibly, he was referring only to the two Indiana survivors, who continued their journey to California. Dils also stated that most of the passengers were from Indiana and that they landed at Kansas City. Again, this is another inconsistent statement, as all other accounts demonstrate that the majority were with the Philadelphia and St. Louis companies, and the *Monroe* was unable to travel any farther than Jefferson City. The article also stated that Dils continued on his journey to California, which is a half truth, as he went home first, got married and then traveled to California at a later date.

One newspaper reported: "From Thursday [May 10], the day the *Monroe* landed at the wharf, until the Sunday evening following, there were 37 deaths; and from Sunday until yesterday evening [May 13], there have been 15, making in all 52 deaths out of about 150 passengers on board the boat. We also learn that several deaths occurred among the passengers who left this city and would not remain with their sick companions."[80]

Interestingly, the cholera was confined primarily to the cabin passengers and some of the Philadelphia and St. Louis company who occupied the hurricane (boiler) deck. Once the steamer was close to Jefferson City, the discrepancies in events start to play out even more clearly. "Phil E. Chappell, a twelve year old at the time who later became a city river merchant, banker and mayor, claimed that residents greeted the Monroe with an old cannon named 'Sacramento.' They threatened to blow the vessel out of the water if it attempted to land. Cooler heads prevailed, he said, and frightened residents eventually allowed the ship to dock at the landing."[81]

The story of the cannon was troubling to me until I read the book *Fire, Pestilence and Death: St. Louis 1849*. In it, Christopher Gordon talks about warnings to boats near St. Louis that they needed to stop for cholera, or health, inspections. Located on a bluff overlooking the Mississippi River at St. Louis, the St. Louis Arsenal was outfitted with "a cannon of proper caliber supplied with cartridges." The objective was for it to fire if a boat hadn't stopped for inspection. This would then alert the officials upriver that a potentially contagious steamer was approaching. "Regulations called for ten rounds to be fired from the cannon as the errant steamboat powered by, clearly making the point that the city meant business."[82]

St. Louis was facing a serious cholera epidemic. On the worst days, there were upwards of 160 deaths, with approximately 10 percent or more of the city's population eventually falling to the deadly disease. No wonder it took extra precautions to be sure all steamers were inspected. Even though Jefferson City never reached epidemic proportions with the cholera, at this time, the cannon "Sacramento" may have been used in a similar way to warn passing steamships. There was no question that Jefferson City wanted to keep itself clean and free of disease. James McHenry remembered:

> *We had no quarantine regulations at that time, but the people were a law unto themselves. As long as the cholera prevailed no steamboat was allowed to land. When a boat arrived in sight of the town the mayor was notified and with a squad of citizens he proceeded to the levee and forbid it to land. The captain's declaration that he had a clean bill of health and that he was subject to a suit for damages for failure to deliver his freight availed nothing, the boat had to move on.*[83]

In Eldon Hattervig's article in the *Missouri Historical Review* about the history of the "Jefferson Landing," he commented:

> *Active commercial traffic encouraged repeated exposure to contagious diseases, such as cholera. Residents anxiously sought to keep out steamers carrying the dreaded disease but hoped to appear humane toward misfortunates. Periodically, Jefferson City newspapers printed denials that cholera had infected the city.*[84]

The preceding accounts go along with the account of Captain James E. Murphy, the clerk and owner of the steamer, who was also on board the *Monroe*. He wrote a letter to the *St. Louis Reveille* printed on May 17 in which he claimed that the ill and dying were treated by the citizens of Jefferson City very inhumanely. He claimed that the citizens left some of the dying "in a vacant house where they died without attention, and others were left to die in an open market house." He also singled out the "keeper of the Missouri House," James Herndon, for closing his doors to all but a few who would pay his outrageous prices.[85] In his letter to the *Reveille*, Murphy failed to mention that, on landing at Jefferson City, he quickly left the steamer and

> *went to a hotel, paid no attention to the sick, and left the same evening in the stage for St. Louis, leaving orders to the clerk not to give up the baggage of those who would not pay their full passage to St. Joseph. This, some of the passengers done, and others refused. Many were left without a thing, unless they remained on the boat, and very few would do this.*[86]

In a letter to the editor of the *Jefferson Inquirer*, Joseph Hammar, one of the ship's survivors, asked:

> *What opportunity had James Murphy to know the treatment which the sick received, when he left on the second day after landing? With what justice does he dispense praise and blame, who left his own hands to be waited upon by the citizens, to be buried by the city? With what grace can he speak of extortion who had not only refused to refund to needy passengers a portion of their fare to towns above here, but even sent to the bedside of the dying who were buried at the expense of their friends, to demand their fare?*[87]

James A. Crump, the original owner of the Lohman building at the southwest corner of Jefferson and Water Streets, opened the "Missouri House" in April 1841. The hotel, located in the upper floors of the building, was advertised as a

> *house for the accommodation of travelers and boarders, in his large Stone Building, at the lower steam boat landing. Near the capitol, where he is prepared to accommodate all who may please to favor him with a call. He has taken considerable pains to arrange his house for the accommodation and comfort of persons travelling on boats. His bar is kept in the basement story, and immediately above he has a large and commodious setting room, in front of which he has erected a portico from which persons can have a beautiful view of the river and can see steam boats 8 or 10 miles up and down. My rooms are large and well furnished, and no pains shall be spared to render satisfaction to all who may favor him with a call. It is expected that the steam Ferry Boat will land at this point during the season and if not, persons putting up with me and wishing to cross the river, shall be crossed without delay, or the fatigue of carrying their baggage to the other landing, nearly half a mile from the business part of town. My stables are convenient, and persons wishing to hire horses, can at all times be accommodated.*[88]

Captain Murphy also "states that some of the English Mormons acknowledged having had sickness among them in St. Louis. Children had died; they had lived together, &c., yet their appearance was sufficiently cleanly on coming on board."[89] This was an incorrect assumption on his part. It appears he didn't know very much about his passengers or where they had come from.

If any of the Philadelphia company had died before their gaining passage on the *Monroe*, it is likely that William Appleby would have recorded that in his journal. He made no mention of such, other than that of Elijah Malin. It is also possible that Captain Murphy was referring to those English passengers who had sailed up the Mississippi on other steamships. Many of them had been afflicted with the cholera, and many of their children probably died. Murphy returned to his home in New Albany, Indiana, arriving on May 20, 1849. He had traveled there on the steamer *Aaron Hart* along with a couple of the Jeffersonville survivors.

The *Aaron Hart* was a 261-ton side-wheel steamer built in Elizabethtown, Pennsylvania, in 1848 for the Pittsburgh–St. Louis run. It was much larger than the *James Monroe*, as the following description shows:

> *The length of her deck is 182 feet; keel 167 feet; beam 27 feet; floor 26 feet; hold 6½ feet. Her hull was built by Mr. B. Coursan, of Elizabeth, and is a substantial and thoroughly finished piece of work.*
>
> *Her "Clipper Engines" were put up by Messrs. Lee & McGinnis. Her cylinders are 16 and 32 inches in diameter, respectively, with six and a half feet stroke.*
>
> *She is provided with two boilers, each 26 feet long, and 42 inches in diameter.*
>
> *The Wheels are 25 feet in diameter with 9½ feet buckets.*
>
> *The Cabin combines all the modern improvements, and was constructed by Mr. Thomas Moffitt: on whose taste and skill it reflects credit. It has 40 state rooms and can comfortably accommodate 82 passengers.*
>
> *The upholstery is from the excellent establishment of Mr. Seibert, Fourth street.*
>
> *The carpets—very fine ones,—are furnished by McClintock; the splendid furniture by R. Fairman of Allegheny; the large and costly mirrors by T.A. Hillier, Wood street; the queensware and lamps by G.R. Massey.*
>
> *The Bell was furnished from the foundry A. Fulton, Fourth street.*
>
> *Her guards, both on the hurricane and boiler decks, are remarkably graceful yet elaborately ornamented with carved work; and her Texas and Pilot House—towering to an unprecedented height above the water—are as much distinguished for their convenient arrangement as for their elegant appearance. The Texas is provided with rooms for all the officers, besides a dining hall, sufficiently large for their accommodation.*[90]

Unfortunately, it was destroyed in a wharf fire in New Orleans in October 1849. The *Hart* was insured for $25,000, but it carried 150 tons of cargo worth about $250,000. There appears to have been only two deaths, that of a cabin boy and a deck passenger.

These records have similar undertones. Several of the accounts of this sad situation specifically state that it was a ship full of "Mormons." If they were familiar with the previous "extermination" order against the Mormons by former governor Lilburn W. Boggs of Missouri (Executive Order 44, issued October 27, 1838), then it is a possibility that both stories were tainted by negative views toward members of the Church of Jesus Christ of Latter-day Saints.

Not surprisingly, neither of the previous accounts mention those who worked on the ship or those from Indiana as having died. It appears that Captain Murphy may have been looking out for his personal interests in the

Monroe; it is also possible that Phil Chappell, as a twelve-year-old lad, was caught up in the excitement, and his prejudice and recollection may have faded as he recorded his experience years later as an adult.

In contrast, there are numerous letters to newspapers, as well as journal entries, that do not agree with the notion of passengers being treated inhumanely. These accounts seem to be more in line with what most likely occurred. They also agree with William Appleby's previous statement that some of the local citizens went on board the *Monroe* to help care for the sick and dying.

In attempting to piece together an accurate telling of the events, with the support of these other accounts, it has been claimed that Captain Moore, immediately on landing, left the boat and found a room at a local hotel. He took no interest in the welfare of his sick, dying or dead crew, nor in the welfare of the passengers. It was said that he left "orders to the clerk [of the *Monroe*] not to give up the baggage of those who would not pay their full passage to St. Joseph."[91]

That evening, he gained passage on a stagecoach back to St. Louis, where he died of the cholera soon after arrival. His death occurred on May 12.[92] It is also possible that some of his traveling companions also died from the cholera before they reached St. Louis.

To gain passage on the stagecoach, Captain Moore would have had to cross the Missouri River on the ferry to the Callaway County side, where the stagecoach ran. "The first ferry license [in Jefferson City] was granted to Wm. Jones. Among the fees he was allowed to charge was, 'For single men 18 ¾ cents.' That was right enough, but as nothing was said of married men, it is hoped, in considerations of domestic hardships, that they passed free, and perhaps were not allowed to pass at all."[93]

Directly north of the wharf, in Callaway County, was the property of John Yount and the destination of the ferry.

On December 21, 1836, the First Session of the Ninth Missouri General Assembly approved the Jefferson Ferry:

> *Act to authorize James A. Crump and others to keep a Ferry at the city of Jefferson.*
>
> *§ 1. James A Crump, James Logan, and John W. Wells, are hereby authorized to keep a public ferry across the Missouri river, within the limits of the City of Jefferson, free from license for fifteen years from and after the first day of September next, and shall have the exclusive right and privilege of keeping a ferry within the aforesaid limits of the city aforesaid: Provided,*

That the said Crump, Logan and Wells, shall on or before the first day of September next, furnish a good and sufficient boat to be propelled by steam power, and well furnished with the necessary engineer and hands to attend the said boat, to be used in crossing the said river, as a public ferry, within the limits aforesaid, and keep the same in repair.

§ 2. The said Crump, Logan and Wells, shall, to entitle themselves to the security, in a sum to be determined by the county court of the county of Cole, conditioned for the faithful performance of their duties under this act, which bond shall be approved by the court aforesaid, and filed with the clerk of said court.

§ 3. The said county; court of Cole county, shall, and it is herby authorized and required to regulate the ferriage across said river, from time to time, as the same may be deemed proper.

§ 4. The said Crump, Logan and Wells, and their securities, shall be liable upon their bond aforesaid, to any persons who may suffer damage, by detention or otherwise, in crossing said ferry, and the same may be sued on by any person aggrieved, and a copy of the same, under the seal of the court, attested by the clerk, shall be sufficient evidence in any trial for damage as aforesaid.

§ 5. If said steam boat shall burst its boiler, or otherwise get out of repair, said proprietors shall have the same repaired as speedily as can be done, and shall, in the meantime, procure and keep such other boats as will be sufficient to do the ferrying at the said ferry.

§ 6. It shall be the duty of the said company hereby incorporated, at all times to transport, over the river persons on foot, persons on horseback, wagons and teams, and stock of every description, to and from the landing on the north side of the river, above the mouth of Cedar creek, and a failure to do so, shall be deemed a violation of this charter; and the rates of ferriage shall, in no case, for services contemplated by this section, be higher than for like services in transportation to and from the north side of the river below the mouth of said Cedar creek.

§ 7. It shall be the duty of said company, at all times, to keep the banks at the places of landing in as good repair as the nature of the banks will permit, that wagons and passengers of every description may pass with safety.

§ 8. If said county court should be satisfied that said proprietors have failed to comply with any of the provisions of this charter, they shall have full power to establish other ferries as they may think proper, in conformity to the general law, for the time being.

> *§ 9. Said Crump, Logan and Wells, shall land all passengers, who require it, as near the centre of population in said city, as the stage of the water will permit.*
>
> *§ 10. Said charter shall not affect the rights of persons owning lands to the water's edge.*
>
> *§ 11. This act shall not be so construed as to authorize the said Crump, Wells and Logan, to ferry from the opposite shore, without a license from the county court of callaway county.*[94]

On February 11, 1839, this "Act" was amended in Section 1 to "James A. Crump, Enos B. Cordell, John Yount and Jefferson T. Rogers"[95] as being the ones authorized to keep a ferry. "The first steam ferries were owned and run in 1839 by Jeff. T. Rogers, E.B. Cordell, T.L. Price, and John Yount."[96]

Over the years, the wharf at Jefferson City had gone by various names, including Rogers Landing, Yount's Landing, Jefferson Landing and Lohman's Landing. By October 1848, a new steam ferryboat had been placed in operation by J.T. Rogers, running from the wharf at Jefferson City to the opposite shore in Callaway County. "He has procured good and substantial floats, or landing boats, and horses, wagons, &c., may at all times cross the river with ease and security, and in the short time of two minutes and a half."[97] The ferry at Jefferson City was the only ferry within forty or fifty miles, so it was critical for providing access to the state capital.

There is truth to the fact that the citizens of Jefferson City were afraid of the cholera. Jefferson City had been disease-free and had been working hard to make sure it stayed clean. Unfortunately, no one fully understood the cholera, how it was contracted or how to treat it. Many still felt it was a contagious disease, despite doctors assuring the public of the opposite.

The *Jefferson Inquirer* stated: "In the evening [May 10] the boat dropped below the city and tied up."[98] Another report stated: "At first the wharfmaster would not let the boat land. It turned back down the river for a mile where it docked and passengers got off and walked back to Jefferson City."[99] And according to another report, "The mayor and aldermen forced the boat and its passengers to relocate below the city."[100] This account fits with the mayor, Jefferson T. Rogers, having called a "meeting of the Board of Aldermen" on May 11 (the day after the landing), after which they "procured a comfortable building in which the sick were to be placed."[101]

John Yount, the owner of Lohman's Landing, where the *Monroe* first docked, tried but was unsuccessful in keeping the steamer from "tying up."[102]

Many of the citizens, panic-stricken at the thought of the cholera being on their shores, closed their doors and refused to assist the passengers. This was not an unexpected reaction.

Dr. George Bickerton Winston, one of the physicians who cared for the cholera victims, was known in his day as one of the most well-respected physicians in the county. In later years, he was asked, "Doctor, what necessity is there for this ceaseless labor and study at your time of life?"

His response provides a good look into his character and how he may have considered his responsibility to care for those victims.

> *My dear sir, I am under bonds to do it. When I offered my professional services to this community there was an implied covenant on my part, so far as God gave me strength and ability, I would use them for gathering up and digesting all that has been said or written in regard to the diseases to which human flesh is heir, and if I should lose a patient because of my ignorance of the latest and best experience of others in the treatment of a given case, a just God would hold me responsible for the loss, through inexcusable ignorance, of a precious life, and punish me accordingly; and whenever I get my consent to be content with present professional attainments and trust to my own experience for success, I will withdraw from the practice and step from under a weight of honorable obligation which with my best endeavors to meet honesty and conscientiously, still sometimes is almost heavier than I can bear.*[103]

I believe that Dr. Winston's words demonstrate that at least the doctors in the city took great care in their interactions with the cholera patients.

Downstream from Lohman's Landing about a mile or so was the Missouri State Penitentiary. Just to the east of the penitentiary, at the end of Chestnut Street, was the prison landing, where the *Monroe* could have been removed to. It landed there or just tied up along the shore near there. Appleby recorded in his journal that by nightfall on the day of the steamer's landing (May 10), it had been removed to near the prison. This date is inconsistent with the date of May 11, when the local Board of Aldermen met.

The idea that a wharf would not allow a steamer to land is not unique to Jefferson City. Just before the *Monroe* left St. Louis, the steamer *Mary*, also bound for Council Bluffs, had departed from St. Louis. When it approached St. Joseph, Missouri, the residents of that town gathered at the Missouri River to try to prevent not only the steamer from landing but also the unloading of its freight. Between St. Louis and Council Bluffs, the *Mary*

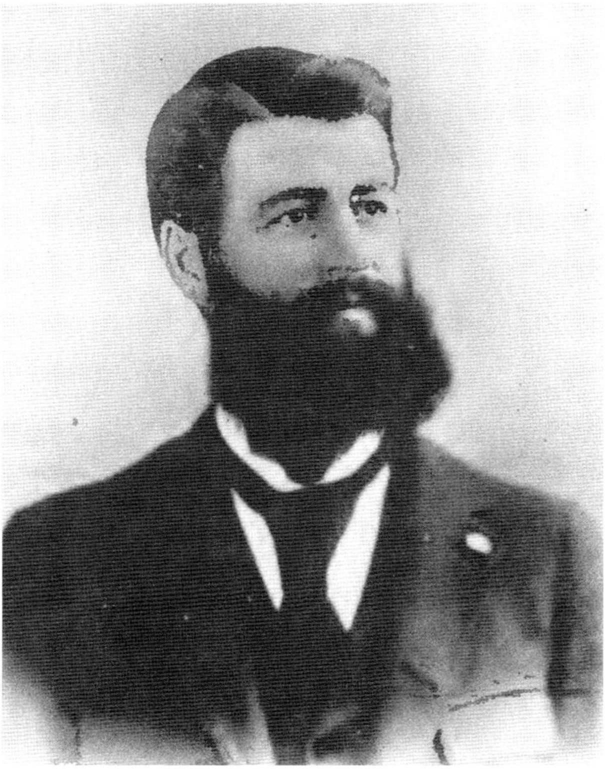

Dr. George Bickerton Winston. From *The Illustrated Sketch Book and Directory of Jefferson City and Cole County*, 1900. *Library of Congress.*

lost about 15 percent of its passengers to the cholera. Most of its passengers were Welsh immigrants.[104]

The only thing the passengers of the *Monroe* could do was look for medical help for the ill and dying and lodging for themselves. Captain James Murphy stated that many tried to find lodging in the Missouri House. "Some of them encamped on the river bank,"[105] while others just laid down on the bank, near where the *James Monroe* was docked, waiting for the most likely fate of death. Others found lodging in the "Virginia Hotel"[106] (the landlord was John D. Currey) and in several of the large vacant houses in town. These houses were vacant because their owners had left to pursue gold-digging in California.

It was said that John Currey of the Virginia Hotel would allow boarders from the steamer to stay for only two nights and one day, at which point he ordered them to leave, his reason being that if they stayed any longer he was afraid he would lose his regular boarders. He also confiscated their mules to help pay for their lodging. A mule cost about five dollars, a lot of money for two nights and one day. I am not sure whether the members of the Church had many animals, but those men from Indiana did. It was also reported that Currey wouldn't even help the sick obtain water to drink. After the panic subsided and the local citizens heard of Currey's behavior, the locals became more generous in helping the sick and the dying.[107]

The Virginia Hotel was a large brick building located near the corner of Jefferson and High Streets. It contained twenty-four large furnished rooms available for borders and other patrons. It even had a bar on-site that carried a large choice of the best liquors.

Dr. Davidson, one of the attending physicians for the cholera victims, wrote, "On the arrival of the boat, so great was the panic, that, for the first few days, no assistance was rendered in nursing."[108] His sad account fits with the idea of the dead and dying lying along the bank in the cold rain. No one fully understood the cholera or what to do about it. One can't know if the number of deaths would have been lower had medical care been provided sooner.

Because Jefferson City had no hospital at that time, several makeshift hospitals were created to care for the ill and dying. One home that may have served as a hospital was the Gustavus Parsons House, located at 105 Jackson Street. This home is still standing today. It is said that it was used as a hospital during the 1849 cholera epidemic, but I am not sure if it was used at this time or later in the year.

With the suggestion of Judge James W. Morrow, and under the direction of local parishioner and vestryman Dr. William A. Davison Sr., the Episcopal church, located on the east side of Madison Street near the corner of East Main Street (now Capitol Avenue), directly across from the Madison House Hotel, was converted into a makeshift hospital. The church was built in 1842 as a two-story stone building.

Additionally, the Presbyterian church was also converted into a makeshift hospital. The one-room stone building was erected about 1844. It was located on the south side of Main Street, directly across from where the Governor's Mansion was at that time. Main Street was later renamed Capitol Avenue, and the long-gone church building would now be in the parking lot of the Governor's Office Building. Also, the old Methodist church was said to have been used to care for the sick. I am not sure whether this church (located on the south side of Main Street between Madison and Monroe) was used to care for the *Monroe* patients or if it was used later in the year. To be used as hospitals, the churches' benches had to be removed and straw mattresses placed on the floors for the sick and dying to lie on.

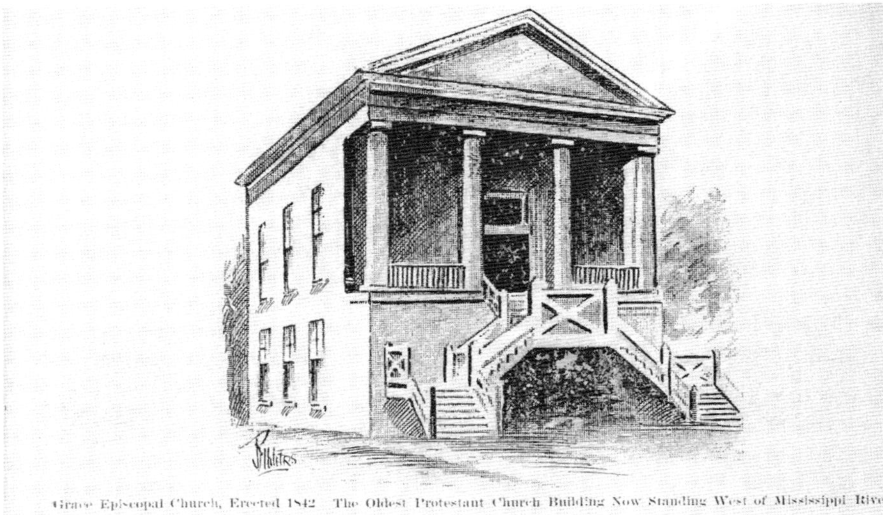

Above: Grace Episcopal Church, erected in 1842. From *The Illustrated Sketch Book and Directory of Jefferson City and Cole County*, 1900. *Library of Congress*.

Opposite: Presbyterian church in 1844. *First Presbyterian Church*.

The White House (an unoccupied hotel) was also used as a hospital. In 1840, the White House Hotel was "fitted up in a most excellent style, for the accommodation of travelers and boarders.…The White House is situated on Main street immediately in front of the Capitol and the lower steam boat landing,"[109] at the southwest corner of Main and Jefferson Streets.

In January 1842, the White House, owned by H. Rea, caught on fire and, fortunately, was not completely destroyed, despite the city having no organized fire department. "By unprecedented exertion, however, the house was saved, with very considerable injury. Think of this! A house saved after being wrapped in flames, without the help of engine, ladder, fire hooks or fire company! At some future time, we believe our city authority, intend providing means for the extinguishment of fire!!!"[110]

I am not sure if it was rebuilt, but this could help explain why it may have been unoccupied.

Interestingly, all of the buildings used to care for the victims were very close to each other. It was only one block up Jefferson Street to Main Street, and the buildings used as hospitals were only about a block to the east. Even the hotels many of the passengers found lodging in were close by.

First Presbyterian Church, Jefferson City, Missouri

Church Buildings Through the Years

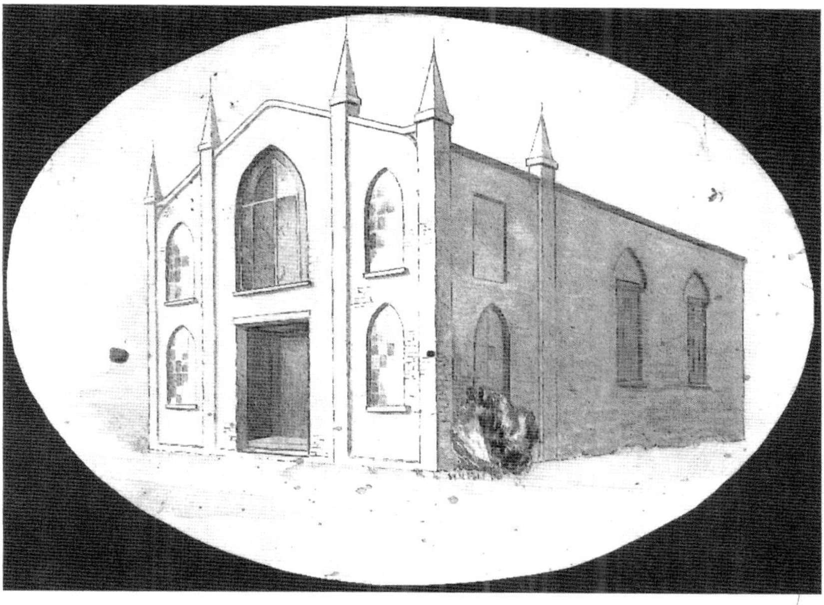

First Presbyterian Church Building in Jefferson City, Missouri 1844. This one-room building was constructed by the Presbyterian congregation on a lot on the south side of Main Street, across the street from the executive mansion of that period. The street later was renamed Capitol Avenue following construction of the new state house to replace the capitol that burned in 1911. Location of this church building, if still standing, would place it in the parking lot of the Governor Office Building in 2002. Last use of the building that could be found in records was as a carpentry shop.

Hospital care would have been very primitive for those suffering. An account from the City Hospital in St. Louis describing care (in general) said: "Patients typically lay on straw mattresses on the floor, rather than in beds, and aside from the resident physician, there was nothing that resembles professional staff. Nursing was provided by local women who were often recruited, it was said, by local policemen who recommended women whom they knew from their daily beats. In the evening, the nursing staff went home, and a night watchman was left to provide care."[111]

There is also the account of Presley Cordell, who said, "It is a difficult matter to get any one to nurse the sick, which has probably been the cause of more deaths than would have otherwise occurred."[112]

The quality of care for those suffering in Jefferson City was likely similar to that described in a newspaper report: "The negroes only asked the modest sum of $5 and $10 per night for nursing them."[113] William Appleby observed: "Nurses were hired, and paid as high as three dollars per day, and others five dollars per night, for attendance on the sick, besides Doctors Bills, which were high, besides three dollars for digging a grave, and from six to nine dollars (I believe) for a common pine Box or Coffin for the dead."[114]

Fourteen-year-old James Edgar McHenry recorded that he worked as an errand boy for the sick in the Episcopal church, gathering soap and medicine as needed. Other boys also helped by carrying ice to the patients.

Additionally, we have the account of Judge Charles L. Wells, who wrote in a letter dated May 12:

> *Two of the churches, some of the hotels, and three or four vacant houses and many tents are filled with the sick besides those at the boat, which now lies near the house of Gov. Edwards, just below the city. The corporation employs all the nurses and attendants which money will procure. The funerals are generally, I believe, at the public expense. I know not the number of cases now on hand; I was informed that one physician prescribed to-day for 32 or 33.*[115]

Judge Wells also said that, by 5:00 p.m. on the twelfth, he had observed seventeen burials that day. Additionally, he said that, since the steamer had docked, thirty-three passengers and crew had died. There is some confusion regarding his statement about the residence of Governor Edwards. John C. Edwards was the former governor and had traveled to California soon after his term was up in November 1848. Wells may have had him confused with the current governor, Austin Augustus King.

In 1849, the Governor's Mansion was located at the northwest corner of Main and Madison Streets. If that is the location where he observed the *Monroe*, it places the steamer at or near the landing at the end of Jefferson Street, another possible conflict in the story.

Many local physicians assisted in caring for the sick. Dr. William Armstrong Davison Sr. (age thirty-nine) studied medicine at the University of Pennsylvania, When he moved to Jefferson City, he worked in partnership with his brother Dr. Alexander McDonald Davison. He was known for being kind and generous, with a pleasing and gentle disposition.

Dr. Alexander McDonald Davison (thirty-six), the younger brother of Dr. William Armstrong Davison, also studied medicine at the University of Pennsylvania. He was known for his medical ethics and his lack of tolerance for those who didn't live up to them. Alexander Davison was known to have spent many days caring for the *Monroe* cholera victims when he did not remove his clothes at night, only to catch a few short hours of sleep in his stable.

Dr. John Henry Edwards (forty-three) was a partner with Dr. Rufus Abbot. "He was a resident of this city for twenty-five years or more; was a most popular and successful physician, had a large and lucrative practice, and by his gentle demeanor and kind attention to all whom he was called to visit professionally, he became personally as well as professionally a universal favorite in the circle of his practice. He was a plain, unassuming man, caring nothing for show and parade."[116]

Dr. Alexander Pope Dorriss (thirty-one) studied medicine with Dr. Abbot before attending the St. Louis Medical College. "He was kind, generous, unselfish, and never did harm wilfully to any living creature. He was sociable, hospitable, charitable, never turning the hungry from his door unfed, nor the needy unaided, to the extent of his ability. The fountains of his cheerfulness never failed, but rippled on through prosperity and adversity the same, bringing light, and warmth, and sunshine to his own heart and to all with whom he came in contact."[117]

A German immigrant, Dr. Ludwig H.A. Krause (thirty-one) had received his medical training in Germany.

Dr. George Bickerton Winston (twenty-seven) was a graduate of McDowell Medical College in St. Louis. He was the first president of the 1873 Medical Society of Central Missouri and was very active in civic affairs, including having served as school board president.

James E. McHenry remembered in later years a Dr. Wm. Abbott, but I have not been able to confirm that name. The only William Abbott I

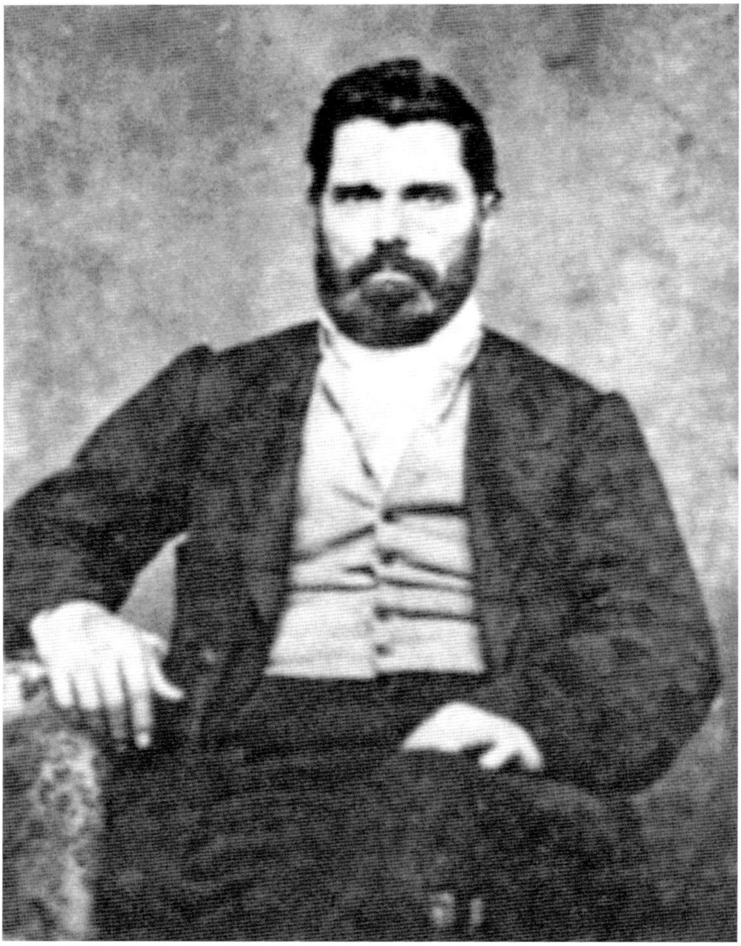

Dr. Tennessee Matthews. *Janice Fry.*

found was a farmer. I did, however, find a Dr. Rufus D. Abbot (forty-two) practicing in the Jefferson City area at the time. He was living in Callaway County. Dr. Abbot had mentored Dr. Alexander Pope Dorriss. He also worked in partnership with Dr. John H. Edwards. In 1865, he was appointed superintendent of the Missouri State Lunatic Asylum in Fulton. "He was a learned, judicious and successful physician—one in whom contemporary physicians, as well as the people, reposed great confidence. He was decided in his opinions, firm in executing his designs, and punctual in the discharge of his duties."[118]

Most of the care Dr. Abbot provided to the sick he did without any consideration for payment. It was said that none of the local doctors provided a bill to any of the cholera patients unless one was asked for.

As a graduate of the Louisville Medical College, Dr. Tennessee Matthews (thirty-nine) spent over thirty-three years practicing medicine in Cole and its adjoining counties. In addition to working as a doctor in Jefferson City, he also served as mayor, alderman, coroner, justice of the peace, president of the Jefferson City Volunteer Fire Department and city magistrate. Additionally, he operated the Tennessee Hotel and the City Drug Store, located in the 100 block of East High Street.

Dr. Richard Allen Wells was twenty-nine years old. A Dr. Richard Alexander Wells served in the Civil War from Jefferson City. I believe they are the same individual.

Additional doctors named who helped care for the victims included Dr. H.D. Linn (twenty-four) and Dr. William Adams Curry (twenty-two). There may have been more, but all the doctors mentioned here were known to have been directly involved in the care of cholera victims.

When one looks at the character of each of the physicians who cared for the *Monroe* victims, it is easy to see that they possessed high principles regarding the care of others. Unfortunately, not all reports confirmed this standard of ethics. One unsubstantiated report in the *New York Evening Post* was as follows:

> *One Doctor D*[aviso]*n here must have made $1000 in ten days. His first question, after looking at the tongue, was to inquire of the state of the purse. His modest fee was usually $100; take all the cash the poor fellow had, or his mule and plunder, then take his note for remainder.*
>
> *Dellinger, Of the Indiana emigrants, lay in his bed, supposed past recovery, when a fireman from* [the] *Monroe came into his room and commenced rifling his pockets. Poor D. yelled, but to no effect, the rascal took out $100 in gold and vamosed. D., in his excitement, jumped out of bed and gave alarm; the fellow was pursued, caught and is now in jail. He denies the charge, and they can get no money from him. Dellinger recovered.*[119]

Another description of what appears to be of the same account said:

> *While lying between life and death, with the living and the dead almost indistinguishable from each other lying around him, that a sacriligious* [sic] *thief paid his visit to the place to strip the dead and the dying of what they*

had in the way of money or valuables. Coming to Dellinger he found him alive but heeding not in the least, and remarking with brutal coolness that it could be of no use to the owner, he proceeded to rifle his pockets and left him with only $4 in shinplaster.[120]

The rest of this sad plundering tale was that Dellinger, now recovered and penniless, was desirous to return home.

In this evil plight he fell in with a Louisville captain and to him he told his tale. To the everlasting credit of this truly humane man be it said that the worst of Dellinger's trouble vanished when he met him. Having heard his story this captain agreed to take him back with him to Louisville for the scanty remuneration which was all he could offer—$4 in shinplaster. On these terms Mr. Dellinger returned to the old home but the captain's generosity received but scant reward, for the shinplasters he found unable to turn into useful commodities and he may have the credit of carrying his passenger free of charge.[121]

A shinplaster was a common name for paper money of low denomination circulating widely in the frontier economies of the 19th century. These notes were in various places issued by banks, merchants, wealthy individuals and associations, either as banknotes, or circulating IOUs. They were often a variety of token intended to alleviate a shortage of small change in growing frontier regions. They were sometimes used in company shop economies or peonages in place of legal tender.

Shinplasters circulated in the United States from 1837 to 1863, during the period known as the "Free Banking Period." According to the Oxford English Dictionary, the name comes from the quality of the paper, which was so cheap that with a bit of starch it could be used to make papier-mâché-like plasters to go under socks and warm shins.[122]

Supporting the hope that the citizens of Jefferson City treated the cholera victims better than some of the previous accounts lead one to believe, there is the letter to the *Jefferson Inquirer* written by several survivors (Charles Foster, Henry Delinger, Wm. E. Lafferty, R.R. Rmter (Ruter), R.M. Pincham, John W. Hampton and Joseph Hammer):

If individual instances of extortion have occurred, though we know of none such, nothing certainly can compare with the conduct of this Jas. Murphy, clerk and owner of the boat. Who brings accusations against the people of this town, and who in the whole affair, has seemed to be actuated by a desire to make the utmost out of the trip, without regard to truth, honor, or the lives of those under his care. His boat crowded through his misrepresentations as to the number of passengers; foul and freshly painted, as the coats of the passengers and physicians here will testify; the berths illy ventilated, and the mattresses in such a condition that some preferred to take blankets and sleep on the hurricane deck, justify this assertion.[123]

On May 14, 1849, Presley Thomas Cordell Jr., a local resident, wrote a letter to his father in St. Louis in which he said that thirty to forty deaths occurred among the passengers and crew since the boat landed. He said that on the fourteenth, four bodies were buried with three or four more ready to die. He was in Boonville, Missouri, when the steamer landed and did not return to Jefferson City until a few days after, but he recognized the sick and dying as needing immediate care and wrote:

As soon as I got back I went to work nursing the sick. A just many appear to be afraid to go near them; but what could I do? The sick were perfect strangers here, without friends and in just need of attention. I do not profess to have greater courage than others, but, with a firm and humble reliance on the protection of Divine Providence, I have watched by them in the night, administering medicines and doing the best in my power to relieve their sufferings, endeavoring to following the golden rule, to do unto others as I would have others do unto me.[124]

He also wrote that he was not aware of a single case of cholera affecting the local residents. It was also said that "our Physicians never inquired or presented a bill, unless asked for it by a friend of some deceased person."[125]

Another firsthand experience was recorded in 1893 by James Edgar McHenry. As a fourteen-year-old lad in 1849, he regularly went down to the Missouri River to watch for boats. He was surprised to see the *James Monroe* lying at the wharf with no steam and no sign of anyone on board. All he could see were passengers and their baggage lying on the levee, with all of the passengers looking sad and distressed. He had heard that after the *Monroe* had landed, the captain and several of the crew deserted the steamer and went across the river to find their way back to their homes.

In an example of his faded memory, he stated that the steamer *Timour* was the ship that carried the cholera. This was unlikely, as the *Timour* was one of the steamships that burned in the tragic wharf fire in St. Louis on May 17, 1849. However, there was a *Timour* (no. 2) that traveled regularly through Jefferson City, possibly later in the year. Unfortunately, it met its fate, destroyed when all three of its boilers exploded while it was docked at Edwards' wood yard just below the penitentiary on August 26, 1854, at about 2:00 p.m. The entire forward part of the steamer was destroyed, causing the hull to sink toward the upper deck. Approximately fifteen individuals were killed, and five or six others were wounded.

Those who stayed behind in Jefferson City included F.W. Peters, the ship's second clerk, and the mate, John J. King.[126] What eventually happened to them, I do not know. A few days later, McHenry ventured from his home on the south side of Main Street, across from the Missouri State Information Center building erected in the 1990s, to downtown. He was surprised to find everything looking deserted. He saw no one visiting the local businesses and no horses or wagons on the streets. Only a few individuals, gathered in small groups, were talking quietly and looking afraid and anxious. The only businesses that were busy were the saloons, also known as groceries, because they carried the food staples a family would need.

He remembered only seventy-five passengers being on board, with only two surviving. He also stated that most of them were California migrants. This is an incorrect observation, since approximately thirty-five on board were from Indiana, bound for California, while the majority (approximately one hundred) were members of the Church of Jesus Christ of Latter-day Saints from Philadelphia and St. Louis, bound for Council Bluffs. This is much more than the seventy-five passengers he remembered.

One of the sad consequences of a disease such as the cholera attacking a large group of people is the death of children. Cholera usually attacked the elderly and weak first, then children second, with the mothers (who cared for the children) being third. The strong and healthy were usually the last ones to become ill. Because several children were left without parents, the public administrator, Captain Mosby Monroe Parsons, became involved. He took possession of the money and property of the children's parents until a friend or family member could claim it. Several small children were known to have returned to Philadelphia, but it is unknown whom they traveled with.

A mystery of this fatal illness is, where were the dead buried? One account says that "the graves of her passengers ranged along the shore for about a half a mile."[127]

Edward Sayers wrote a letter to the editor of the *Inquirer*: "We were, sitting all night in a drenching rain, with no other covering than night clothes,—some lying prostrate, others in the agony of death—graves digging by our sides, and the departed being put into them, can only be felt by those who were actually there."[128]

Then there is this account: "They were buried near the place of their death."[129] Here is another such report: "They fill the strangers' grave on the banks of the Missouri."[130]

Appleby recorded that he "visited the Boat [relocated to near the penitentiary] from time to time, to seek after our goods. The sick and dying—graves side by side, coffins on the shore. Beds, and pillows, half burned sick beds etc. which the sick had lain and died. Bedquilts, Blankets etc. were floating around the shore, and down the river together with, Broken Pots, Jugs, Bowls, strewed along the Banks of the River, all, all had a tendency to add to the mournful scene."[131]

These accounts tell us that the weather was rainy, probably cold, and that graves were being dug by the side of the dying. All of this happened at night. Since the *Monroe* was moved to near the prison before nightfall, these accounts could imply that graves were dug "by their sides" on the bank of the Missouri River near the prison. W.I. Appleby wrote a letter to the editor of the *Frontier Guardian* in which he said, "And to add to the horrid spectacle were the graves, side by side—beds and pillows half burned up—pieces of tents, broken cups, bowls, pillows, matrasses, &c., lined as it were the banks of the river, near the boat; while blankets, mattrasses [*sic*], beds, &c, on which the sick had died came floating down the river; while in town, nothing could be seen scarcely but carts and hearses loaded with rough coffins (chiefly)."[132]

Interestingly, Appleby talks of seeing graves along the bank near the relocated boat by the penitentiary and not downtown near the Lohman Building. He also separates the location of the graves from "in town."

Then there is the newspaper account that states "that a death trench from the site of the building [Lohman's Landing] to the present Missouri Pacific Railroad station contains most of the graves."[133] Another one claims that "victims were buried in a trench dug downstream near the site of the present Missouri Pacific Railroad depot."[134] This statement, which implies that the dead were buried in a trench, references the May 19, 1849 edition of the *Jefferson Inquirer*, which is partially incorrect. Nowhere in that paper is a trench mentioned. It did, however, state, "We can assure the friends of those who sleep in our grave yard that no pains were spared to save them from the grasp of death."[135]

The idea of a "trench" being dug to bury the dead fits with the description of what happened in St. Louis. The city was hit much harder with deaths from the cholera; over four thousand died of that dreaded disease. One account says: "Every morning the 'dead wagon' made its round, accompanied by the awful cry 'bring out your dead.' Accompanying these wagons were immunes who would enter, take the corpses, sometimes without any preparation, to the vehicles, and then on to the cemetery where, due to the heavy death toll, the corpses were buried in trenches, hundreds at a time."[136]

Another example of misinformation was contained in a 1960 newspaper article: "When the Mormons were coming into Missouri to settle near Independence in 1848, cholera broke out on the boat after it left St. Louis. All the passengers were unloaded at Lohman's Landing and it was used as a hospital. Sixty-five who died were buried in a single grave."[137]

First, it was 1849 and not 1848, and the boat was not headed for Independence as a final destination. Also, this is the only reference I have found that Lohman's Landing was used as a hospital during the epidemic, which doesn't fit other accounts telling of John Yount, the proprietor of Lohman's Landing, trying to prevent passengers from debarking at the wharf. In addition, the reference to everyone being unloaded at Lohman's Landing is inconsistent with other accounts that tell of passengers still on the steamer after it was relocated downstream to near the prison. However, the reference to all of the victims being buried in a single grave fits with the concept of a "death trench" where the dead were interred.

Then there is this report: "The work of death went on. The tramp to the grave-yard was almost constant."[138] Additionally, Phil E. Chappell wrote: "The boat stopped about a mile below town, and the poor unfortunate passengers, in their effort to escape from the plague-ridden vessel, came up the bank of the river, where many of their dead bodies were found."[139]

There are some discrepancies among these numerous accounts. Several accounts tell of the dead being buried where they died, while others talk of hearses constantly transporting bodies to their place of burial. This, of course, could be referring to bodies being carried from the hospitals or other places of death.

There were also reports of a quarantine area. Henry Dellinger remembered that "the health officers quarantined them and they were taken ashore and isolated."[140] The news also reported: "The official authorities of Jefferson City have declared that place in a state of quarantine, and no boat is permitted to land without undergoing a scrutinizing search."[141]

We also find the following report: "The steamers Amelia and Monroe [were] at Jefferson city, lying up. The authorities of that place have established a quarantine, and boats are not permitted to land without first being inspected by a committee of physicians."[142]

Also on May 13, the City of Jefferson Board of Aldermen met and introduced a bill that established an ordinance (1849–12) for a quarantine area to be located within the center town tract. Since it was required that a bill be read three times before it was voted on, the bill was read three times during the meeting, approved and then immediately signed by the mayor. Also at that time, Dr. Alexander Pope Dorriss (one of the physicians who cared for the ill and dying) was appointed as the health officer for the city. A quarantine area established within the "center town tract" fits well with the location of the makeshift hospitals and hotels where most of the victims were housed or cared for.

The 151-ton side-wheel steamer *Amelia* was built in St. Louis in 1846 by Emerson for a cost of around $12,000. It was owned in Jefferson City and named for Amelia Cordell. "The *Amelia* was laid up at Jefferson City" because of low prices and the scarcity of freight.[143] It sank near Glasgow, Missouri, in December 1849.

I can see four possible locations for the burial of the victims.

1. By the evening of the day the steamer landed, it was removed to near the penitentiary. Possibly, the dead were buried near its relocation. This would fit with the accounts that tell of the dead being buried at night near where they died and the reference to coffins laying along the shore. The penitentiary location would have been in an area not as highly populated by visitors to the city and would not have had a rock bluff to contend with. This location could also have had the use of prisoners as laborers to dig a trench. "The History of Cole County" also states that the *Monroe* "landed all her passengers below the city, where sixty-three died and were buried."[144] That one statement lends a great deal of support to the penitentiary area being the location for the burials.

2. If there was a so-called trench, or even a mass grave, dug near Water Street, it is questionable where it would have been dug. To dig it to the south of Water Street would have put it into the rock bluff. In between would have put it in the middle of the narrow dirt roadway known as Water Street; in addition, the bedrock is not very deep, so an adequate trench would have been extremely difficult to dig. Additionally, I do not

believe that city officials would have wanted a burial site in such visual proximity to where visitors and commercial traffic entered the city from the river. Another issue is that if you go too far north, you place the trench on the property of the Missouri Pacific Railroad. Even though the railroad was not built for several years, the land would most likely have already been purchased and surveyed.

3. Another possibility is that they were buried in a mass grave somewhere else in the city, such as in the Old City Cemetery. If this was the case, there is no known record of it having happened. Several accounts talk of hearses running constantly, carrying coffins with the dead in them. People who were sick were moved to a place for care, such as the makeshift hospitals, a hotel or one of the vacant homes in the city. No one would want the sick and dying to lie for too long in the open for all to see and smell. No matter where the victims were buried, hearses would have had to transport the coffins from the place of death to the place of burial. The first possibility places the burials outside of the quarantine area and in a less-populated place. The second possibility places the graves within the city quarantine area. The third possibility also has the burials outside of the quarantine area. I'm not sure how transporting the bodies through the streets of the city would have been received, but in all three scenarios, transporting bodies would have been necessary. The problem with this third possible location is that a report states, "They fill the strangers' grave on the banks of the Missouri."[145]

4. The fourth possibility is that because the first to die were brought ashore at the city wharf before any of the churches were turned into hospitals, and because others died after the *Monroe* was moved, it may be possible that there was more than one burial place for the unfortunate victims.

James Edgar McHenry recorded in 1893:

> *When the citizens learned of the situation they organized and took charge of the sick, turned all the churches, the courthouse and vacant houses into hospitals and gave the dead and dying all the attention possible. After a few days my scare subsided and I ventured uptown—we lived at the foot of Richmond Hill, on Main Street. I found it a deserted, desolated looking village. The streets were white with lime, and tar was burning everywhere filling the air with its odor. There was no business doing in the stores, no*

wagons on the streets, and but few people, and they were gathered in little squads talking low and looking scared and anxious. The only places doing any business were the "grocerys" as saloons were called. The good citizens could be frequently seen passing in and out of these "doggeries." It required a great deal of red whisky and hot brandy to keep the cholera at respectful distance from the average citizen in those trying times. At least it made that impression on my youthful mind.[146]

There was the widespread belief that if one burned barrels of tar, the black smoke would clear the air of the cholera. Some people burned vats of lime to help fumigate the air.

On June 4, the Board of Aldermen met and adopted a resolution that invited anyone who had claims for "services rendered the sick during the late sickness from Cholera" to present their claims to the "Committee on Claims." This notice was written on handbills posted in the "most Public places in the City."[147]

At the July 4 board meeting, several claims against the Corporation (the City of Jefferson) for services rendered were presented. Among those individuals were:

Herman H. Wagmann, $7.50, allowed $0.50.
John Harry Bolton, $6.00, rejected.
Elijah Ramsey, $4.00, rejected.
James B. McHenry, $12.00, rejected.
C.L. And William D. Meredith, $36.00, rejected.
Thomas Lawson Price, $24.75, rejected.
John Grieshammer, $14.50, offered $1.50.
George W. Bolton, $5.50, offered $1.00.
Dr. Alexander Pope Dorriss, $7.50, offered $7.50.
James Lusk (for Ramsey), $1.50, offered $1.50.[148]

It had been said that men from all walks of life helped with caring for the cholera victims. In 1849, Thomas Lawson Price was elected the eighth lieutenant governor of Missouri. Previously, he had been chosen as the first mayor of the City of Jefferson. He was known to have been involved in caring for the sick.

Over the next several months, there were numerous accounts of other individuals dying of the cholera in the area. Gaining an accurate account of the number of victims is virtually impossible, as many deaths were not reported through the newspapers. The cholera appears to have reached the area by traveling up the Mississippi River to St. Louis and then up the Missouri River. We have the following report: "The steamboat *Timour* [No. 2] carried cholera to Jefferson City later in 1849. It broke out in the village of Westphalia that summer, taking the lives of one-third of the population."[149]

6
THE CHOLERA

Cholera was known as the "Disease of the 19th Century," making its first known appearance in the Americas in 1832. The symptoms of cholera, which are very similar to those of acute arsenic poisoning, begin with diarrhea, acute spasmodic vomiting and painful cramps. The "disease loosened the bowels and let loose gushes of what was called ricewater stool (the floating white specks were bits of lining from the small intestine). The explosive diarrhea was followed by a hurling up of the contents of the stomach. Patients' eyes sank into their heads; their skin turned leathery, their lips bluish."[150]

There were also distortions of the entire body, including the face and the skin of the forehead. Usually, these symptoms were accompanied by dehydration, with cyanosis and a blue and pinched face, as well as cold and darkened extremities and hands and feet drawn and puckered. In most cases, the pulse could not be felt and respiration almost completely stopped. Dr. McCormick of the United States Army tells us:

> *Cholera has four distinctly marked stages:*
>
> *1. Loose dejections.*
>
> *2. Watery discharges by the stomach, bowels and skins.*
>
> *3. Corpse like coldness, and blueness of the skin, or collapse.*
>
> *4. Reaction, Choleric fever, a state strongly resembling Typhus.*
>
> *The first consists in a simple looseness of the bowels—the defections being frequent and more or less copious and thin, the consistence decreasing*

with each evacuation until it arrives at the next plainly marked stage of the disease. The second period—the evacuations now consist of little else than a watery fluid. With these discharges the thirst is always intense and the voice begins to fall. The stomach becomes involved, pouring forth the same watery fluid in greater or lesser abundance, and ushered in with this evacuation from the stomach, bowels, and skin, and apparently intimately connected with it, is seen the most painfully distressing phenomena of the terrific malady, the cramps and spasms, causing the patient at times to writhe in agony, giving forth every expression of pain that human torture could provoke.

The third period follows, and consists of collapse. This seems naturally explained by the waste of the watery portion of the blood, and the great exhaustion of the nervous system, so intimately connected with it, and with the violent cramps and spasms. The voice has become more feeble, the watery evacuations cease, the agony is over, for the spasms have also ceased, and the patient lies indifferent, apathetic, fearless, and craves only drink. The thirst continues intense, becomes insatiable, and seems to exist in a direct ratio to the quantity of watery fluid poured forth by the discharges, and to depend thereon. It seems to arise from an instinctively desire and urgent demand to supply the waste and drainage of the system. The whole body shrinks, the features become contracted, pointed, peculiar, (Chronic countenance,) the eyes deeply sunken in their sockets, balls rolled upwards or natural, expressing great suffering or total indifference. The skin is as cold as a corpse, and moist, of a bluish hued, varying in intensity of color and extent of surface it occupies; the hands and feet, particularly are so shriveled and corrugated, and greatly shrunken, having lost at least one third of their bulk, and look macerated in water, (like a wash woman's hand;) the pulse is scarcely discernible or extinct, and the action of the heart feeble; the air enters the lungs, but respiration is laborious, with a sense of suffocation from the changed conditions of the blood, that prevents the full vivifying influences of the air on it—the passivity being such that it does not flow in its usual channels, which expose so great a surface to the action of the air throughout its minute and abundant capillaries. The voice enfeebled and greatly diminished, has become husky and nearly extinct, and the demand it makes is still for cold drinks, ice water. They complain of being parched, burning up, and yet the whole surface is icy cold, and possess an exalted sensibility, sinapisms, blisters, &c., are loudly complained of burning like fire—insupportable, even the hand of a healthy person, brought in contact with a collapsed Cholera patient, I have heard loudly complained of as burning. The tongue is cold, broad, flat and dry, or mucous and pasty—the abdomen retracted. In short the whole body has become collapsed. The blood changed, in its character, deprived of its watery portion, no longer traverses its accustomed rounds, but collects in the heart and veins, especially the larger trunks, in undue quantity. The change of place, arising from a change in the passivity of the blood, gives rise in its turn to other changes. There is no arterial blood—there is no secretion, perhaps, except that of bile, for as before stated, the blood has forsaken the arteries, and retreated into the veins.

Throughout all this frightful havoc of the physical frame, the mind moves calmly, clearly, self possessed, and begins to feel the destructive influence, or is gone (with but few exceptions) only when the brain has ceased to be supplied with aerated blood—only when the individual is in articule mortis [point of death].

The fourth state seldom occurs. But when an individual becomes collapsed and lives through it, the fourth stage is present—it is one of reaction, resembling typhus.[151]

Death usually occurred within a few hours to a day from the first occurrence of symptoms. All of the symptoms occurred with little or no warning. "Most of the unfortunate victims died of cardiovascular collapse, usually because of acute dehydration and marked electrolytic imbalance; multiple bleedings by the physicians most likely shortened the life expectancy in some of those victims, already in a precarious, abnormal, fluid imbalance."[152]

The 1849 worldwide cholera epidemic was said to have started in India in 1848 and was brought to this country through such ports as New York, Baltimore and New Orleans. The latter was critical, because many foreigners traveled up the Mississippi to St. Louis, bringing the cholera with them.

For a long time, many doctors believed that cholera was caused by bad air, or "miasmic vapors," that resulted from the odors of decaying garbage and waste. Other theories involved victims eating "excitable" foods such as sauerkraut and ripe vegetables. Some believed that beer and other forms of alcohol were the cause. One theory even suggested that imbalances in the human body were caused by a high number of thunderstorms, thus triggering the cholera.

The cholera usually attacked suddenly, without warning. An individual could be fine one minute, and the next, he could be suffering from severe symptoms. After an incubation period of one to three days, symptoms, which included a sudden attack of painful diarrhea with recurring vomiting, surfaced. Diarrhea was usually marked by profuse watery stools amounting to three to four gallons a day. Then dehydration became critical, along with painful cramping and eventual circulatory collapse. As a result of the circulatory symptoms, the patient would then develop a bluish coloring of the skin because of a lack of oxygen entering the blood. His face would then appear gaunt and hollow-eyed, followed by hands and feet becoming cold and contorted. The cramping was often so painful that the patient often would writhe on the floor in anguish. If a patient went untreated, the fatality rate was about 50 percent.

Some of those who did survive were left with the possibility of long-term side effects, especially issues with the kidneys. The cholera was not selective in its victims, but usually, healthier, robust individuals found themselves spared from the more acute form of the disease. "Malnutrition, intestinal parasites, or other chronic disease conditions made a person more susceptible to the disease. Insufficient food, combined with inadequate sanitation, represented the greatest factor that led to serious outbreaks among Mormon immigrants at sea."[153]

I am not sure of all the differences, but it was reported that there were five different kinds of cholera: cholera, Asiatic cholera, cholera asphyxia, cholera infantum and cholera morbus.[154] Several newspaper reports of the period refer to the *Monroe* as carrying the Asiatic cholera. AudioEnglish.org defines the various types of cholera this way: Cholera is "an acute intestinal infection caused by ingestion of contaminated water or food."

Asiatic cholera is defined identically.

Cholera infantum is "an often fatal form of gastroenteritis occurring in children; not true cholera but having similar symptoms."

Cholera morbus is "severe gastroenteritis of unknown etiology; characterized by severe colic and vomiting and diarrhea."[155]

Cholera asphyxia "is an aggravation of all the symptoms. The icy coldness of the tongue, the blueness of the whole surface, the attenuated, shriveled state of the palms of the hands and soles of the feet, all bespeak nature in the last verge of existence."[156] This is when the victim becomes unconscious because of oxygen starvation during the third stage of the cholera. Very few individuals survive this third stage.

Treating cholera was hit or miss. Some doctors recommended a weekly bath, keeping out of the night air and retiring to bed early. Others said to avoid vegetables and, when that made no difference, to avoid meat. The same went for alcohol; some said to drink it, while others said to abstain from it. Home remedies such as putting mustard seed in one's shoes were also prevalent.

Drugs containing such ingredients as "calomel, laudanum, opium, camphor, capsicum, and spirits of ammonia"[157] were routinely used. Additionally, some physicians believed in bloodletting, vein injections, cautering and cutting the carotid artery in the throat. Even "the use of camomile [*sic*] tea, tobacco and port wine"[158] was recommended.

Unfortunately, the death rate was often higher when patients were treated with these remedies. Some were even given rhubarb to counteract the toxic effects of the high doses of drugs they were given. Young James McHenry remembered that, after having seen the deserted steamer with its passengers being scattered on the levee, along with their baggage, he hurried home, where he "took a good swallow out of mother's camphor bottle as a preventative, having heard somehow that that was the proper thing to do under such circumstances. For a long time I attributed my escape from the disease to that dose of camphor and a few others clandestinely taken."[159]

In 1849, the Committee on Hygiene in Paris, France, released a report of its opinions on the treatment of the cholera.

> *Cholera is not contagious, and it is important that this fact should be thoroughly understood.*
>
> *During the prevalence of the epidemic, the collection of the sick into narrow damp, badly ventilated situations, greatly favor its intensity and extension. Persons attacked in the situations should be instantly removed.*
>
> *During epidemic* [conditions,] *cholera derangements of the digestive functions are more common.*
>
> *1. Those who feel symptoms of colic or diarrhea, or who have pains of the stomach, should be excessively prudent in diet; and avoid fatigue, cold, and humidity. They should wrap the abdomen in a flannel jacket, go otherwise warmly clad, and use mild infusion of tea, or sage, or chamomile, or balm.*
>
> *If these symptoms do not suddenly disappear, a physician should be sent for.*
>
> *It rarely occurs that attacks of cholera are not ushered in by symptoms of disease of the stomach and bowels. In this condition any intelligent person is capable of giving relief; and promptitude is the important point.*
>
> *2. If the disease is not checked in* [t]*his, its first stage—and if diarrhea increases, accompanied with vomiting, chilliness, coldness of the extremities—the patient must be placed in a warm bed, between blankets; have hot bricks, or bags of sand, or bottles of water, applied to his feet, and warm napkins to the abdomen and stomach—the extremities must be*

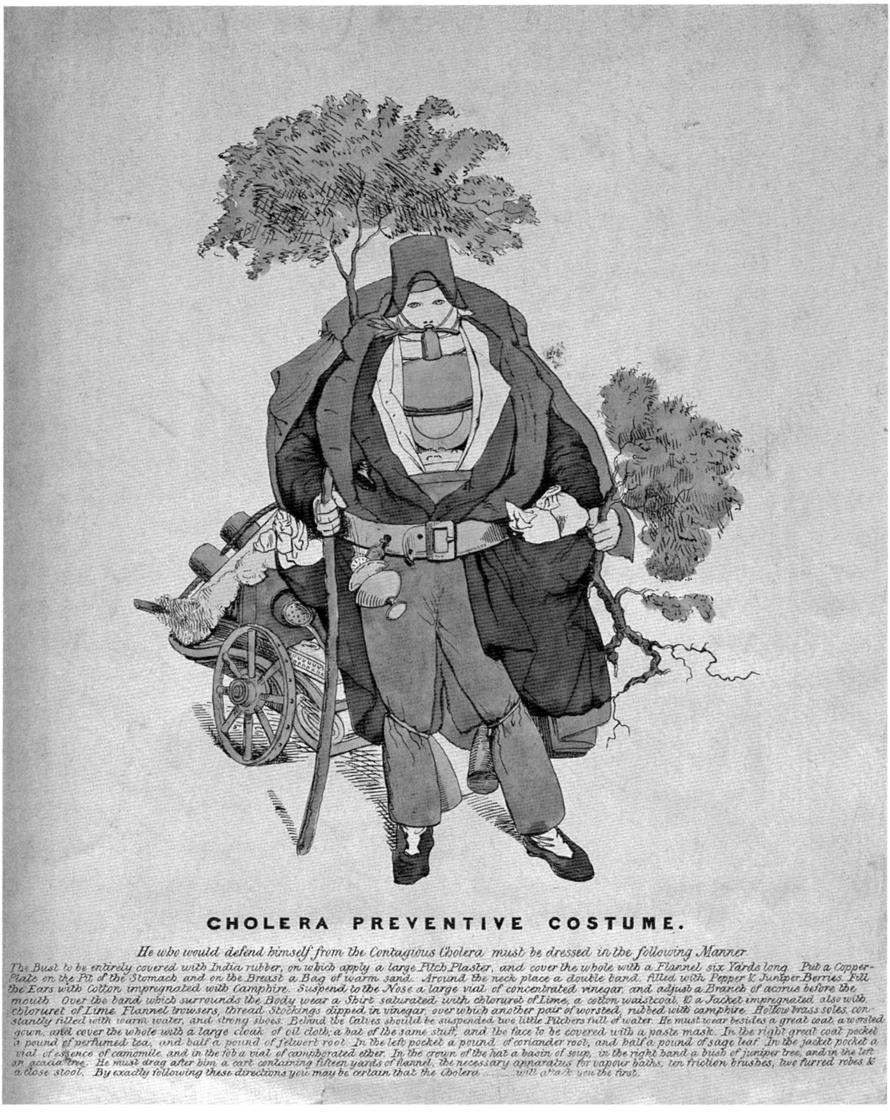
CHOLERA PREVENTIVE COSTUME.
He who would defend himself from the Contagious Cholera must be dressed in the following Manner
The Bust to be entirely covered with India rubber, on which apply a large Pitch Plaster, and cover the whole with a Flannel six Yards long. Put a Copper-Plate on the Pit of the Stomach and on the Breast a Bag of warm sand. Around the neck place a double band, filled with Pepper & Juniper Berries. Fill the Ears with Cotton impregnated with Camphire. Suspend to the Nose a large vial of concentrated vinegar, and adjust a Branch of acorus before the mouth. Over the band which surrounds the Body wear a Shirt saturated with chloruret of Lime, a cotton waistcoat, & a Jacket impregnated also with chloruret of Lime. Flannel trowsers, thread Stockings dipped in vinegar, over which another pair of worsted, rubbed with camphire. Hollow brass soles, constantly filled with warm water, and strong shoes. Behind the Calves should be suspended two little Pitchers full of water. He must wear besides a great coat, a worsted gown, and cover the whole with a large cloak of oil cloth; a hat of the same stuff, and the face to be covered with a paste mask. In the right great coat pocket a pound of perfumed tea, and half a pound of felwort root. In the left pocket a pound of coriander root, and half a pound of sage leaf. In the jacket pocket a vial of essence of camomile, and in the fob a vial of camphorated ether. In the crown of the hat a basin of soup, in the right hand a bush of juniper tree, and in the left an acacia tree. He must drag after him a cart containing fifteen yards of flannel, the necessary apparatus for vapour baths, ten friction brushes, two furred robes & a close stool. By exactly following these directions you may be certain that the Cholera .... will attack you the first.

Colored etching of a figure dressed in a cholera safety suit, 1832, by J. Petzl. *Welcome Library*.

> *rubbed with flannel dipped in alcohol, camphor, or other stimulant—warm drinks must be administered every few minutes; such as teas, chamomile, &c.—cataplasms of ground flaxseed and mustard must be put on the extremities—all causes of chilliness must be avoided—and small injections of rice water, starch, or decoction of poppy heads superadded—frequent small injections are best.*
>
> *3. When pains in the head, cramps in the limbs, and extension of cold occur—when the tongue is cold, the eyes sunken, the skin bluish on the face and hands—the remedies above indicated should be more promptly used until a physician arrives.*
>
> *Those who apply these remedies must not be discouraged if immediate relief does not follow. A considerable time frequently elapses before a decided impression is made. After this stage of the disease the Committee deem further direction, unless, as none but a physician is capable of comprehending what should be done.*[160]

What was the cause of the cholera on the steamer *Monroe*? That's a question one can only speculate on. Indeed, the cholera was making its way up the Mississippi River from New Orleans, or down the Ohio River from Pittsburgh, but some of the speculations were that "the sickness was mostly attributed, by the Physicians, to the newly painting of the boat, and the emigrants using the Missouri River water, which they were unaccustomed to."[161] Additionally, it was said that the passengers could readily detect the strong smell of the lead paint (the paint being still wet), coupled with inadequate ventilation. This could have played a role in the contracting of the cholera. It was also said that (referring to the steamer *Consignee*), "the crowded passenger quarters and ignorance of sanitation provided grimly ideal conditions for the spread of cholera."[162]

Another report said that those seeking passage on the boiler deck of the *Monroe* "piled their baggage up very high, and spreading a canvas over it, entirely excluded air from that quarter of the boat. The heat in the cabin, over-crowded and freshly painted, was insufferable and almost unendurable during meal times. Every cheek paled beneath this dreadful atmosphere."[163]

No wonder deck passage was cheaper, but also not as healthy. "Often the lower deck passengers received no food or drink, except for river water. They were obliged to work for their passage alongside the roustabouts and to find a place to sleep amongst the cargo, exposed to the weather. If cots were provided, it was likely they harbored lice or some contagious disease, making the woodpile or stacked cargo a more inviting place to sleep."[164]

Physicians have also said "that the disease spreads among the deck passengers. Very few cases are ever reported by the cabin passengers. The cleaner cabin decks may account for this difference."[165] This is an interesting observation that seems to fit the deaths by the cholera on other steamers. It was unusual to find just the opposite occurring on the *Monroe*, where most of the victims were lodging in the cabins. This tends to support the theory that the paint and the ventilation were contributing factors in the spreading of the disease.

There is also an account of a

> *gentleman from Boston who spent the winter in New Orleans and recently came up the River, who say's that in all the cases where cabin passengers were attacked, the Cholera yielded to prompt treatment and nursing. But that steerage passengers as soon as taken, were laid in a small exposed place, back of the wheelhouse, and though in many cases the disease was checked, yet nearly every sick man died from a lapse produced by exposure. The answer of the clerk when appealed to, to place them in a more comfortable position, was that he could not put them in the cabin, they had been driven out of the steerage, and he could give them no better spot than the one they had.*[166]

What follows is another interesting theory:

> *The suspicion that Kreosote may be beneficial in this disease is strengthened by the facts stated in your paper of Friday:—that while many persons had sickened and died suddenly of this disease on board the steamer Monroe at Jefferson city, Mo., "not a death had occurred on the deck of the ill-fated boat"—that all the sickness had been confined to the cabin "passengers, and some who occupied the boiler deck." It is well known that deck passengers on the western steamboats are much annoyed with smoke; and might not the inhalation of that impart a quality to the blood which counteracted the tendency of the cholera matter to disturb or destroy the weak chemical combination of the blood.*
>
> *If the effect of Kreosote upon the system when thus inhaled be known, it would be safe to expose small quantities of it for evaporation in the chambers of the sick, it may, perhaps, be a powerful for good, as the subtler and more inappreciable, if not feebler matter, or condition of matter, inducing the cholera, is for evil.*[167]

At the time of the landing of the *James Monroe*, Jefferson City considered itself a very healthy community. There had been several cases of possible cholera, but none of them was contracted within the city before the steamer arrived. It was said that "some ten or twelve cases of Cholera have occurred in Jefferson City, some of which proved fatal. Mr. Henry P. Paulsel, of the 'Paulsel House' in that place died of it on the 18th [April]. Two or three servants have likewise died of the same disease. None of the cases it is said originated in the city."[168]

Another case was that of Dr. Wilson Brown, the auditor of public accounts. He arrived from Cape Girardeau several weeks before the *Monroe* landed. It was said that one or two of the "negroes" on board the steamer with Dr. Brown were sick and died with the cholera a few days after their arrival in Jefferson City. Dr. Brown survived. Another citizen had visited St. Louis before dying locally of the cholera. None of these individuals contracted the cholera locally.[169]

Another death, taken from the journals of William Swain as he traveled the Missouri River, was described in his account of April 28, when he wrote: "Having taken on an extremely heavy lading, we left Jefferson City at two o'clock and proceeded slowly on our way, having on board a company of emigrants from that city. Here we heard of a man dying of cholera."[170]

It was also recorded that "up to this time [May 19] but two deaths have occurred among our citizens of this fearful maledy [*sic*]—one a colored woman, and a Mr. Ruff, a stone cutter."[171] Contrastingly, the *New Orleans Crescent* reported: "*twenty-five* citizens of the generous citizens perished by the fell disease."[172]

James E. McHenry also recounted that "but few of the citizens were attacked. The only one who died, as I remember, was Presley Thomas Cordell."[173] Cordell died on July 28, 1849, in Jefferson City of the cholera. Because his death occurred over two months after the landing of the *Monroe*, it is questionable whether his death was directly related to the cholera on the steamer. How many more local deaths were attributed to the steamer is unknown, but there is no doubt that the cholera had arrived in the vicinity before the *Monroe*'s landing.

In March 1849, it was reported that Richard Fry, an Irishman of strong conviction who was a prisoner at the Missouri Penitentiary, died of the cholera.[174] He was the only recorded prisoner to die of this cause in 1849. His contracting of the cholera could not have been linked to anyone on board the *Monroe*, since he died about two months before its landing.

There doesn't appear to have been any exact records of the number of cholera deaths in Jefferson City during this outbreak, which lasted about two years. Even the local newspapers were silent on many of the deaths. Since the cholera had already attacked several citizens before the landing of the *Monroe*, and since physicians were emphasizing that the cholera was not contagious, possibly only a few of the local deaths were directly related to those victims on the steamer.

Interestingly, none of the physicians who attended to the sick and dying was known to have contracted the disease; only Dr. Stephenson, who attended to the sick on board the *Monroe*, contracted the disease.

7
WHAT NEXT?

The steamer *Lightfoot* left St. Louis at 1:00 a.m. on May 15 with about 110 members of the Church of Jesus Christ of Latter-day Saints, primarily from England and Scotland, on board. On the way to Jefferson City, 7 immigrants who died of the cholera were buried. The *Lightfoot* arrived at Jefferson City on May 16, where approximately 25 passengers from the Farnum and Appleby companies joined them, and left Jefferson City on the seventeenth.

Another report says that 40 of the survivors gained passage on the *Lightfoot*, with all but one of them dying on the way to Council Bluffs.[175] I have been able to identify 37 individuals who made it all the way to Council Bluffs and eventually to the Salt Lake Valley. This number does not include the 2 children born after arriving there. In July, William Appleby wrote to the *Frontier Guardian*, reporting that 160 "Saints" were on board the *Lightfoot* while it was "on the Missouri River."[176]

If 110 passengers left St. Louis on the *Lightfoot* and 7 died before it arrived at Jefferson City,[177] that would leave 103 passengers on board when it reached Jefferson City. After the *Lightfoot* left Jefferson City, there were two known births among the Farnham and Appleby companies, along with several deaths attributed to the cholera. That leaves upward of 50 additional passengers gaining passage on the *Lightfoot* at Jefferson City. It is a reasonable estimate that 40 to 50 additional passengers boarded the *Lightfoot* at Jefferson City.

With the names of twenty-two known dead (including two who had died before reaching Jefferson City); at least eight members of the Church returning to either St. Louis or Philadelphia; at least two individuals and two or three families staying in Jefferson City for a time; the two Hand children, whose final destination is unknown; and the thirty-seven known survivors on the *Lightfoot*, that would leave between forty-four and forty-six known survivors of the approximately one hundred who boarded the *Monroe* at St. Louis. This would mean that about fifty-two to fifty-four individuals from the original Church companies could have died with the cholera between St. Louis and Jefferson City, or approximately half of the original number.

William Appleby made "a contract with Capt. Brooks [of the *Lightfoot*] to convey those of our company desirous of going to the Bluffs, his charges being the same from there as from St. Louis, i.e. $12, cabin, $5, deck, and 62½ cts. per hundred for freight—those of the company not going in the cabin to have the use of the boiler deck, with the offer of given my wife, (as is customary, I being agent of the company) a free passage in the cabin."[178]

Those passengers who survived made it to Council Bluffs, Iowa. Unfortunately, it was not on the steamer *Lightfoot*. As early as Saint Joseph, Missouri, Captain Brooks tried to confiscate the belongings and expel the passengers. When the steamer approached Iowa Point, Missouri, it encountered very high water with a current that was too strong for the steamship to handle; therefore, the captain turned the *Lightfoot* around and traveled downstream to Savannah Landing, about twenty-five miles north of St. Joseph. It was there that the captain forced everyone off his ship, along with all their freight, and secured passage on the steamer *St. Croix* to take them the rest of the way.

Not every member of the Philadelphia and St. Louis companies continued their journey to Council Bluffs. Several of the survivors, who were not members of the Church, returned to their homes in Philadelphia. Likewise, several returned to St. Louis. The names of many of these survivors are unknown. There is the statement that Anne Elizabeth Holman Wilson wrote in a letter to Sister (Mary) Webster on January 1, 1850, in which she said, "some of the company came back."[179]

Anne was living in St. Louis at the time but was unable to travel with her friends and fellow Church members, due in part to illness. She was the sister of Emily Jennison Holman Lewis, who did travel with her family on the *Monroe*. Emily and her family continued their journey to the Salt Lake Valley. Anne Wilson followed in 1856 but, sadly, along with her young son, was killed by Indians somewhere in Nebraska.

As for the Jeffersonville company, only two or three were reported to have continued their journey to California for that rush of gold they so desired. Two of those who continued their journey were Henry L. Dellinger and William E. Lafferty. Additionally, E.S. Dils and Uriah Edwards traveled on to California, but only after first returning to Indiana. The rest returned to their homes in Indiana or other states (such as Kentucky or Ohio). They began their journey with about thirty-five men traveling to California; eighteen were known to have died (several having died before the steamer was forced to land at Jefferson City). That leaves possibly fifteen survivors out of approximately thirty-five who would have returned to their homes.

8
SURVIVORS

Disasters often bring hidden results. One tends to feel sorrow for those who died, but what about those who survived and are left behind, many times alone? Many of them go through periods of severe stress or depression. They are also in need of our concern and prayers.

Determining who survived the cholera on the steamer *Monroe* is no easy task. There was no known ship manifest listing the names of all of the passengers. Newspaper reports were very sketchy about listing those who had survived and those who had died. Many times, an individual was listed as deceased, only for it to be revealed later that they survived. William I. Appleby and R.R. Ruter are two examples of those incorrectly listed as having died. This list of survivors is compiled from multiple sources and contains some suppositions I have made. This list may not be complete, but it does provide a good representation of the survivors.

Unknown daughter (about age twelve) of William A. Adams from Philadelphia survived.[180] Several newspaper articles tell of a William D. Adams of Philadelphia who, along with his wife and his oldest and infant children, died at Jefferson City. **William D. Adams** (age thirty-five to forty) is listed as a member of the Philadelphia Branch of the Church of Jesus Christ, along with his wife, **Elizabeth**, and daughters **Emma Elizabeth** (one) and **Hester Ann** (three).[181] I believe this is the correct William Adams who was with the Philadelphia company. His oldest daughter would have been **Sarah Jane** (sixteen). She could have been mistaken for the twelve-year-old daughter reported having survived.

Unfortunately, the newspaper articles are mistaken when they tell of at least two children dying, as his daughter Emma Elizabeth also survived. Of course, dying does not necessarily mean they finally succumbed to the disease. Emma Elizabeth died in Pennsylvania in 1930. Sarah Jane died in Pennsylvania in 1916.[182] The two surviving girls would have returned to Pennsylvania, but I'm unsure of whom they would have traveled with. Several others returned to Philadelphia, so they could have traveled with any one of them.

William Ivins Appleby (thirty-eight), captain of the Philadelphia company, was accompanied by his seven children: **Augustin** (eighteen), who died in Utah in 1911; **Martha Ann** (fifteen), who died in Utah in 1855; **Curles (Charles) Shimm** (fourteen), who died in Utah in 1898; **William Price** (eleven), who died in Utah in 1918; **Sarah (Sally) Ann** (eight), who died in Utah in 1923; and **Joseph Smith** (three), who died in Utah in 1910.

The older four children were baptized as members of the Church of Jesus Christ of Latter-day Saints on April 9, just before the family left Philadelphia. He also had a daughter **Merinda Ann**, who was born on the steamer *Lightfoot* on June 1, 1849, near St. Joseph, Missouri. She died in Utah in 1926. His wife was **Sarah Brown Price Appleby** (forty). She died in Utah in 1898. They were part of the George A. Smith/Dan Jones Company that left Kanesville, Iowa, on July 14, 1849, bound for the Salt Lake Valley.

William I. Appleby died in Utah in 1870. After arriving in the Salt Lake Valley, he was elected as a member of the First Legislative Assembly for the State of Deseret. He continued in politics and later worked as a clerk for the U.S. Supreme Court in the Territory of Utah. As a young man, he had been trained as a carpenter and millwright. Before he led the company of Church members from Philadelphia, he taught school, had his own scrivener's office and was a county justice of the peace.

Brother Austin of the Philadelphia company. His given name is unknown.

William Darrough Beach (fifty) of Jeffersonville, Indiana, returned home to his wife and children. He died there in 1866. He had worked as a merchant and a salt agent.

George William Bosely was the eight-year-old grandson of **Ann Kelly Bosley**. Because both of his parents had died, he was likely living with his grandmother in Winter Quarters, Nebraska. He would have traveled with her to St. Louis to visit his aunt **Mary Ann Bosley Malin** and uncle **Samuel Malin**. The four of them would have gained passage on the *Monroe* to return to Kanesville, Iowa. With the rest of his family, he joined with the Ezra Taft

Benson Company that left Kanesville on July 15, 1849, bound for Salt Lake Valley. George died in Utah in 1911. He had worked as a cattleman.

Henry Clay Bruner (twenty-two) of Jeffersonville, Indiana, returned home to Indiana to be with his wife and daughter. He died there in 1872. Henry had worked as a ship carpenter and as a farmer.

Henry Logan Dellinger (twenty-four) of Jeffersonville, Indiana. He had been sick with the cholera at Jefferson City. He continued to California. He returned to Jeffersonville about two years later and died there in 1904, apparently as a very wealthy man. Back in Indiana, he had worked as a farmer.

Mr. Detty was from Jeffersonville, Indiana. Unfortunately, I have not been able to determine his first name.

Elias Safford (E.S.) Dils (twenty-five), the son of William and Stokley Dils and the nephew of Dr. William Stephenson, leader of the Jeffersonville company, returned to Indiana. Later, after marrying, he traveled on to California with his wife. Eventually, they returned to Indiana, where he died in 1908. He worked as a farmer.

John C. Eaby (thirty-five) and family of the Philadelphia company, lost his wife, **Eliza Pierce Eaby**, and at least one child to the cholera at Jefferson City. Originating from Lancaster County, Pennsylvania, he continued to Kanesville, Iowa, with his surviving daughter, **Eliza Ann**, age two, where they joined with the Silas Richards Company, leaving Kanesville on July 10, 1849, bound for the Salt Lake Valley. Also traveling in this company was the Augustus Farnham family, which had been on the *Monroe* with them. John Eaby died in Utah in 1900. Eliza Ann died in Utah in 1933. He was known as an honest and upright farmer, respected by all.

Uriah Edwards (thirty-three to thirty-four) of Jeffersonville, Indiana, had been sick with the cholera at Jefferson City. After returning to his home and family in Jeffersonville, Uriah brought his family to Petaluma, Sonoma County, California, most likely in 1850. He died there in 1868. While in Petaluma, he was elected to the state senate and was known as an honest and faithful senator and was a well-respected citizen. At the time of his death, he was serving as the first president of the Society of California Pioneers.[183] To be a member of the organization, one had to have arrived in California before September 9, 1850.

Augustus Alwin Farnham (forty-four) of St. Louis was traveling with his wife, **Mary Jane Pottle Farnham** (thirty-two), and children: **Sarah Mariah Farnham** (four), who died in Utah in 1940; **Mary Jane Farnham** (two), who died in Utah in 1920; and **Ruth Farnham**, born on May 15, 1849, in Jefferson City, Missouri. Ruth died on the way to Utah in 1849.

Anne E. Wilson wrote a letter to Sister (Mary) Webster, dated January 19, 1850, in which she stated, "Br Farnham got a house and took E[mily] and his wife to, where she was delivered of a girl."[184]

Emily Jennison Holman Lewis was known as a midwife in her later years, so assisting in the delivery could have pointed her toward becoming a midwife after she arrived in the Salt Lake Valley. The Farnhams joined with the Silas Richards Company, leaving Kanesville, Iowa, on July 10, 1849, bound for the Salt Lake Valley. Augustus died in Utah in 1865. Augustus was a carpenter by trade. In 1853, he was called to be the mission president of the Australia Mission for the Church. In 1847, the Farnhams had moved to St. Louis, where he was called to be a counselor to Nathaniel H. Felt, the president of the Church there.

Charles Foster of Seville, Ohio, was captain of the Western Reserve Pioneers. Before joining with the Jeffersonville company, Charles had been principal of the Seville Classical School in Seville.

Brother Franklin of the Philadelphia company.

Mr. Graham of the "Jeffersonville Volunteer California Company."[185]

Joseph Hammer (thirty-six) was from Philadelphia. I believe he returned to that city. Joseph was well known to William Appleby, who, in 1847, had blessed his youngest daughter.

John William (Watts) Hampton (thirty-seven) and family from Philadelphia returned there, where his family had begun their journey. Traveling with him would have been his children: **Mary Lamb Hampton** (two), who died in Philadelphia in 1887; **Harriet L. Hampton** (ten), who died in Philadelphia in 1866; **John W. Hampton Jr.** (five), who died in Philadelphia in 1922; and **Benjamin Morgan Hampton** (eight), who died in Philadelphia in 1939. John Hampton and his children had not been baptized as members of the Church of Jesus Christ of Latter-day Saints. John died in Pennsylvania in 1894. John W. Hampton worked as a coal dealer.

Elizabeth Hand, daughter of Elizabeth and William Hand. Elizabeth had been ill with the cholera and was left in Jefferson City; a kind sister and her husband stayed behind to help care for her. Elizabeth was only seventeen or eighteen. By August, Elizabeth, with her brother William, had traveled on to Council Bluffs, where they lodged with their cousin, Albert Merrill. There, Elizabeth met a man by the name of Henry H. Williams. Henry was known as a worthless alcoholic. In December 1849, Elizabeth was married by her cousin Albert Merrill to Henry at Allred Branch, Pottawattamie, Iowa.

Elizabeth and William did not continue with the others to the Salt Lake Valley. In the spring of 1850, they moved to western Missouri. The last that was known of her was her living in Atchison, Kansas, in 1870. The Hands were originally from New Haven, Connecticut.

Another demonstration of the inaccuracies that regularly occur in the newspapers is the account of September 15, 1849: "Miss ELIZABETH HAND, whose parents died here with the cholera, left this place on board the same ill-fated boat 'Monroe,' that landed the family here, destined for the Salt Lake. A few days after her arrival at St. Joseph, she was attacked, as we learn, with something like the cholera, and died very suddenly. She has left a little brother, an orphan, without a relative to take care of him."[186]

This account was posted three months before her marriage to Henry Williams and about a month after she arrived in Council Bluffs.

William Hand Jr. (between ten and twelve) was the son of Elizabeth and William Hand. William stayed with his sister Elizabeth Hand in Jefferson City, then traveled on with her to Council Bluffs. He was living with her after she married, until at least 1850, when they were living in Savannah, Andrew County, Missouri. William possibly died in Missouri about 1865.

John D. Hodges (twenty-one) was from St. Louis. He returned there after the death of his wife, Lavinia. He was not a member of the Church of Jesus Christ of Latter-day Saints.

Emily Jennison Holman Lewis (seventeen), and family, was with the St. Louis company. Emily is listed in a letter from Anne E. Wilson to Mary Webster as having been with Brother Farnham when his wife was "delivered of a girl."[187] Traveling with her would have been her husband, **James Farrell Lewis** (thirty-five), and daughter **Anne Elizabeth Holman Lewis** (one). Emily died in Utah in 1911. James died in Utah in 1898. Anne Elizabeth died in Arizona in 1883.

After reaching Council Bluffs, they joined with the Silas Richards Company, leaving Kanesville, Iowa, on July 10, 1849, bound for the Salt Lake Valley. In December 1849, after arriving in the Salt Lake Valley, Emily gave birth to a daughter, Emily Lewis, who died in Utah in 1883. Emily would have been pregnant with her while traveling on the steamer *Monroe*. Emily was a small woman, barely five feet tall.

James F. Lewis was called to serve a mission for the Church in China. After that, he worked in several positions in local government, serving as a probate judge and as a county commissioner. He was a patriarch in the Church when he died.

J.W. Kerr of the Jeffersonville company.

John J. King was the ship's mate.[188]

William. E. Lafferty (thirty-four) was with the Jeffersonville, Indiana company. He was born in Philadelphia. He continued his journey to California. As early as 1862, he was living in Gold Hill, Nevada. He died in Placerville, El Dorado, California, in 1877, but his residence was Gold Hill. He was known as "a tall, raw-boned Irishman, strong, impatient and unruly. He would take no medicine only as it suited him, and when the cramps seized him he would leave his cot, walk around the room and swear he would neither take medicine nor die. In this manner he wore the cholera out and got well."[189]

Elizabeth Dubois Lamb (twenty-six) was from Philadelphia. After her husband, Benjamin Rush Lamb, died with the cholera at Jefferson City, she continued traveling to the Salt Lake Valley with children **John Isaac Lamb** (six), who died in Utah in 1900, and **Benjamin Rush Lamb Jr.** (two), who died in Utah in 1852. Her daughter, **Elizabeth D. Lamb**, was born at Kanesville, Pottawattamie, Iowa, on September 3, 1849.[190] She died in Utah in 1851. They were part of the Benjamin Hawkins Company that left Kanesville bound for the Salt Lake Valley on June 5, 1850. Elizabeth Lamb died in Utah in 1911. She was known for being an excellent cook and is credited with introducing "Dutch" cheese into Utah. Today, we call it "cottage cheese."

Samuel Malin (thirty-six) would have been traveling with his mother-in-law, Anne Kelly Bosley, and her grandson, George William Bosley. He died in Utah in 1893. His wife, **Mary Ann Bosley Malin** (thirty-three), died in Utah in 1900. William Appleby mentions Samuel Malin in his autobiography and journal as being on the steamer *Lightfoot* with him.

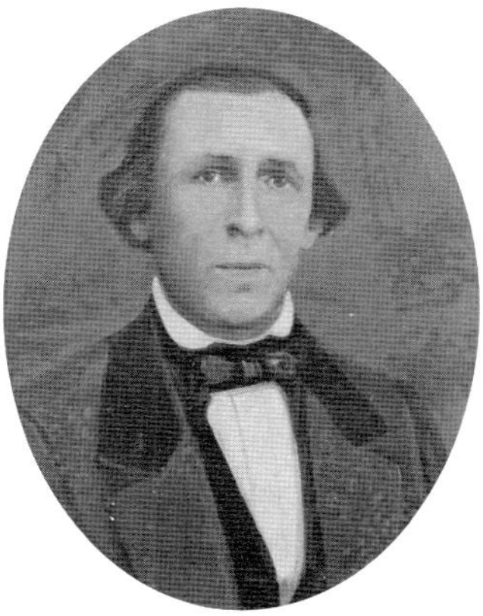

Sketch of Samuel Malin. *David Barton Hansen.*

Additionally, **Council Bluffs Malin**, the child of Mary Ann Bosley Malin, was born on July 1, 1849, at Council Bluffs. He died in Utah in 1942. The whole family was part of the Ezra T. Benson Company that departed Kanesville on July 15, 1849, bound for the Salt Lake Valley. Their original objective was to meet up with Samuel Malin's parents in Council Bluffs to accompany them to the valley. This they eventually did. He worked as a brick mason.

It is probable that **Sarah McGuckin Malin** (forty-six), the widow of Elijah Malin and the sister-in-law of Samuel Malin, accompanied her brother-in-law and his family on the *Monroe*. She is listed on the manifest for the Ezra T. Benson Company along with them. If she was with other members of her extended family, then it is also likely she was accompanied by her children **John McGuckin Malin** (sixteen), **Margaret Ann Malin** (fourteen) and **James Elijah Malin** (ten). John is listed with the Ezra T. Benson Company with his mother; his two siblings are listed as company unknown.

I believe it is likely they all traveled together on the *Monroe* from St. Louis to Jefferson City, and then on the *Lightfoot* headed to Council Bluffs. All of them would have then traveled in the same company to the Salt Lake Valley. Sarah died in Utah in 1877. John McGukin died in Utah in 1896. Margaret Ann died in Utah in 1910. James Elijah died in Utah in 1909.

Captain James E. Murphy was the owner and clerk of the *Monroe*. He returned to his home in New Albany, Indiana.

F.W. Peters was the ship's second clerk.

R.M. Pincham, of Virginia, was with the Indiana company.

Rinaldo Robert (R.R.) Ruter (twenty-one) of New Albany, Indiana, was the son of Reverend Calvin W. Ruter of New Albany. He died in Indiana in 1883.

> *He was a small man, very quiet and patient. After he had been in the hospital several days the doctors pronounced him dead. He was laid out and placed in a coffin, but somehow a spark of life was discovered in him, he was removed from the coffin, revived and nursed back to life and health.… One summer morning in the spring of 1862, during the Civil War, some gentlemen were standing in front of Cloney, Crawford & Company's store, now the Young Grocer Company, when an officer, wearing the uniform of a Federal captain, approached and saluted them. They returned the salute, when the captain said: "Gentlemen, this is Jefferson City, is it not?" They replied that it was. "Things have changed very much since I was here last," he replied. "I had cholera here in 1849, and I died, just around there in the Episcopal church, at least the doctors said I did." Old Captain Vanover, who was in the crowd, spoke out in his usual good natured boisterous way, and said: "Yes, and by the eternal I made your coffin. How are you Captain Rucker* [his correct name was Ruter]. *"*[191]

Cloney, Crawford & Company was a banker and exchange dealer located at the southeast corner of High and Madison Streets. Also, in

1846, William Vanover (born about 1798) was elected coroner in Cole County, Missouri.

It is interesting to note that after returning home, R.R. Ruter attended Asbury College, where he studied to be a physician and surgeon. This was his duty while he served as a captain in Company D of the Eighteenth Regiment of the Indiana Infantry during the Civil War. Maybe the influence for him to study medicine was his relationship with Dr. Stephenson or because of his near-death experience due to the cholera. Asbury College, the original name of Depauw University in Greencastle, Indiana, was founded by his father, Calvin Washington Ruter.

Edward Sayers (forty-seven) was from St. Louis. He was traveling with his wife, **Ruth Daggett Vose Sayers** (forty-one). They were part of the Silas Richards Company that left Kanesville on July 10, 1849, bound for the Salt Lake Valley. The Sayers had previously lived in Boston and therefore were familiar with William Appleby. Edward Sayers died in Utah in 1861. Ruth died in Utah in 1884. According to Anne E. Wilson, Ruth had quite "a time"[192] with the cholera. Luckily, she survived. Edward Sayers was a well-known horticulturist.

J.P. Smith of the Philadelphia company is mentioned in William Appleby's journal. There was a **John Pearson Smith** (thirty-seven) from Philadelphia that Appleby mentions in his journal. He is likely the J.P. Smith that Appleby referred to. He would have been traveling with his wife, **Jane Hart Opdycke Smith** (thirty-four), and his children **Theodore Augustus Smith** (twelve), **Mary Frances Smith** (ten) and **George Opdycke Smith** (seven). They would have stayed in the Kanesville area until their son **Albert Smith** (fourteen) joined them. Albert had left Philadelphia for Burlington, Iowa, early in 1849, staying there through the winter before journeying to Kanesville.

After Albert arrived in Kanesville, and with the birth of John and Jane's son Elwood in October 1850, the family then waited until June 28, 1852, before leaving from Kanesville for the Salt Lake Valley with the Uriah Curtis Company. John P. died in Utah in 1885, Jane H. died there in 1892, as did Theodore A. in 1902. Mary F. died in Nebraska on the way to Utah in 1852. George O. died in Utah in 1902, and Albert died there in 1902. Elwood died in Utah in 1853. John P. had worked as a builder assisting in the construction of the St. George and Logan Temples as well as the Mormon Tabernacle. He was also a charter member of the Tabernacle Choir.

James N. Wathen (eighteen) of Jeffersonville, Indiana, returned there, where he died in 1867. He had been sick with the cholera at Jefferson City. James worked as a boatman.

William Weathers of Jeffersonville, Indiana.

Mr. Williamson, of the Jeffersonville company, was sick with the cholera at Jefferson City.

An **unknown couple** from the Philadelphia company stayed behind in Jefferson City to help care for Elizabeth and William Hand.

There was an additional **one or two families** from the St. Louis or Philadelphia companies who stayed behind in Jefferson City for a time.

Several of the Indiana company survivors returned home instead of continuing their journey to California. They would have arrived home on May 18 or May 19. For those survivors whose final destination is unknown, I believe most, if not all, of them would have returned to their homes.

Lex. Unfortunately, I do not know his full name. Lex could be short for Alexander or Alex. He describes his experience in an "Army Correspondence" he penned to the editor of the *Davenport Daily Gazette* in 1861:

> *Yesterday we left Jefferson City—Before leaving, I visited an old log cabin, where, twelve years since, I spent two weeks under very peculiar circumstances. Some 150 passengers as the steamer Monroe were landed at Jefferson City in June 1849, and in consequence of the cholera the trip was abandoned. Out of one company of six, who were left in the old cabin, the writer alone went out alive at the expiration of ten days. I found also in the city a few old friends, who will always be remembered for their kindness on that occasion, and a letter from Col. Benton to John C. Fremont, (which procured an interview with the family of the latter in St. Louis last month,) as one of the cherished mementoes of the past. Strange, that those who stood by me then, facing, with me, death from terrible pestilence, should now be arrayed in deadly hostility. So it is.*[193]

His description of 150 passengers is consistent with the number of passengers I have suspected. Lex survived the cholera to become part of Company B of the Iowa Regular Infantry Volunteers from Davenport. He may have originated from there. I am not sure if he was traveling with the other five men who were housed in the cabin with him or where they may have hailed from.

9
DEATHS

Just as determining who survived the cholera was no easy task, the same difficulty applies to determining who succumbed to the dreaded disease and died. Through extensive research, I have tried to put a full name to each individual and attempted to verify that they did die of the cholera. This again is not a complete list. I believe there may have been many others, but unfortunately, I have been unable to verify any others.

William A. Adams of Philadelphia died on May 10, 1849. Along with him died his wife and at least one daughter, all on the same day. Several newspaper articles tell of a William D. Adams of Philadelphia who, along with his wife and his oldest and infant children, died at Jefferson City. The newspapers also state that his twelve- or thirteen-year-old daughter survived.

William D. Adams (age between thirty and forty) is listed as a member of the Philadelphia Branch of the Church of Jesus Christ, along with his wife, **Elizabeth**, and daughters **Emma** (one) and **Hester Ann** (three).[194] I believe this is the correct William Adams who was with the Philadelphia company. His oldest daughter would have been **Sarah Jane**, age sixteen. She could have been mistaken for the twelve-year-old daughter who was reported to have survived.

It is my opinion that William D. Adams was counselor to William Appleby. I strongly believe William D. Adams, along with his wife, Elizabeth Adams, and daughter Hester Ann Adams are the ones who died of the cholera on the steamer *Monroe*. There are several discrepancies with the newspaper accounts, as one states that they arrived on the steamer *Mary*,[195] which was traveling from St. Joseph, Missouri, to St. Louis at this time. That would have made it impossible for them to have been on the *Mary*. The whole family is listed in the "Joseph H. McMinn Bible,"[196] with William being listed as having died in Jefferson City on June 12, 1849, of cholera. The month is mistaken, as the newspaper articles all predate that death date.

Additionally, Elizabeth and Hester Ann are both listed as having died on June 12, 1849; another month mistake. The family Bible also tells of only one daughter dying, not two.[197]

Sister Bachelor was from Philadelphia. She died on May 11. W.I. Appleby spelled her name "Batchelor."[198]

Robert Baily, company unknown. Case #37-A of the Cole County Probate records tells of M.M. Parsons, the public administrator, confiscating the properties of "W.D. Adams, Robert Baily, Doctor W. Stevenson, Rice McGrew, William Beach, Davenport, J.C. Edgington, William Edgington and John Edmonson deceased."[199] I am not sure if Baily is the correct surname, but it is my best educated guess.

William Beach, son of William Darrough Beach of Jeffersonville, Indiana, was likely between the ages of fourteen and eighteen.

Ann Kelly Bosley (seventy-one) of the St. Louis company died on May 12, 1849.[200] Ann had been living in Winter Quarters, Nebraska, where her husband died in 1846. She would have traveled to St. Louis with her orphaned grandson, George William Bosley (age eight), to visit with her daughter and son-in-law, Mary Ann and Samuel Malin. Most likely, the whole family accompanied her on the *Monroe* as it traveled from St. Louis to Jefferson City.

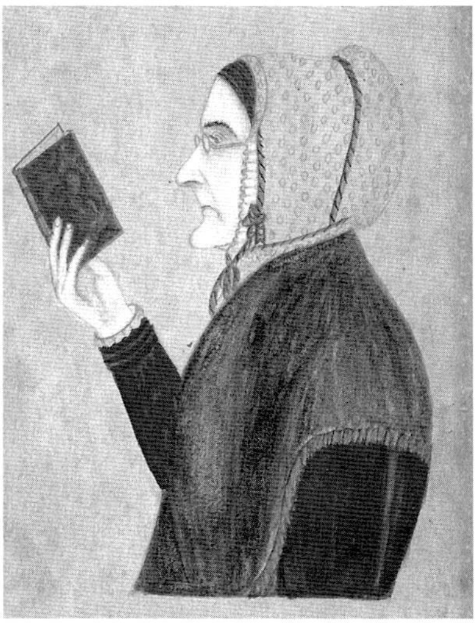

Sketch of Ann Kelly Bosley. *Alan Torbit.*

Her husband, Edmund, is buried in the Winter Quarters Pioneer Cemetery in Winter Quarters. Some have assumed that she was buried next to him, but it is unlikely that her body was transported for several days on a steamship. Most likely, she remained buried somewhere in Jefferson City.

William Appleby tells of a **Sister Boswelle** from St. Louis dying. Since he was not personally familiar with members of the St. Louis company, I believe this may be an incorrect spelling of Ann Kelly Bosley. There was also a reference to "old mother Beckley." I believe that is also a reference to Ann Kelly Bosley. She may have been the oldest individual on the steamship.

Sister Brown of St. Louis.

Mr. Chaflin is assumed to have died along the way between St. Louis and Jefferson City, because he stayed behind when Mr. Williams and Edward McGlenry died and were buried. He most likely would have been with the Jeffersonville company.

James Darrough was from Ohio and was traveling with the Jeffersonville company.

J. Davenport died on May 13. He was with the Jeffersonville company.

Mr. Donsed of Indiana was with the Jeffersonville company.

Sister Eaby was of the Philadelphia company, along with an **unknown child**. I believe she was **Eliza Pierce Eaby** (twenty-nine), the wife of John C. Eaby. They were from Lancaster County, Pennsylvania. One record incorrectly states that she migrated to the Salt Lake Valley in 1848 and died on the trail. William Appleby states, on more than one occasion, that a Sister Eaby and child died at Jefferson City. I am not sure who the unknown child is, as she had two children who may be incorrectly listed as having died in 1848. I believe that one, or both, of them could have died of the cholera with her. That would have been **Jacob Eaby** (five) or **Margaret Eaby** (seven). Her husband and surviving daughter would have continued their journey to the Salt Lake Valley.

Mr. Edgerton of Jeffersonville, Indiana.

William Edgington, a native of Mansfield, Ohio, died on May 11.[201] The son of Thomas Edgington, he was with the Jeffersonville company.

John Edgington, the brother of William Edgington, also of Mansfield, Ohio, died on May 12.[202] He was with the Jeffersonville company.

John Edmonston was of the Jeffersonville company.

Sabra Granger (fifty-five) from St. Louis (also listed as being from Commerce) died on the *Monroe*. As she lay dying, she was attended to by Sister Sayers until she took her last breath.[203] In January 1850, Anne E. Wilson wrote a letter to Sister (Mary) Webster to inform her of the death of Sabra Granger on the *Monroe*: "Appleby's company had a terrible time from beginning to end. They were on the ill-fated (steamboat) Monroe, where the Cholera raged so bad and Aunt Sabra Granger died, she and some other of the Sisters crawled up under the fence and died. The authorities at Jefferson City made all leave the boat, the weather was rainy and windy, some were sick, and some dying."[204]

Hall, gender unknown. Joseph Hammer wrote a letter from Jefferson City to his brother in Philadelphia and recounted the names of several who had died with the cholera. A Hall was listed among those who died.[205]

Sister Mary Jane Hammer of Philadelphia, along with an **unknown child**. They would have been the wife and child of Joseph Hammer, who survived. They died on May 11. A Joseph and Mary Jane Hammer are listed as being baptized as members of the Church in Philadelphia in 1843. They are also shown as having removed their membership from the Church; then they returned, withdrew and were cut off from the Church. It is possible they once again returned to the Church and found themselves in good standing by 1849. Joseph and Mary Jane Hammer had at least two children; the unknown child died with the mother, and an infant daughter (Marinda Hyde Hammer) died previously in Philadelphia in 1848.[206]

Christiana Morris Lamb Hampton (thirty-three), the wife of William Hampton, was from Philadelphia. She succumbed to the cholera on May 10, 1849.[207] She is mentioned as being buried in the Fair Hill Burial Ground in Philadelphia, but I know of no record of a tombstone for her there.[208]

Isaac Lamb Hampton (four) died on May 11, 1849. The son of Christiana Morris Lamb and William Hampton, he is mentioned in the Fair Hill Burial Ground in Philadelphia, but I have found no record of a tombstone for him there.[209]

William Hand (between forty-four and forty-nine) was not a member of the Church of Jesus Christ of Latter-day Saints. He and his family were from New Haven, Connecticut. His desire was to be baptized as a member of the Church once he reached the Salt Lake Valley. His wife, **Elizabeth Ann Merrill Hand** (between thirty-seven and forty-four), also died, along with an adopted son, **Charles Smith Hand** (sixteen), the son of Caroline Smith (deceased).

Lavinia Price Hodges (seventeen), wife of John Hodges of St. Louis. Her husband survived.

John Hubbard (thirty), principal of the Bowling Green Academy in Bowling Green, Missouri, was never heard from again. He died on May 15.[210] John, originally from Massachusetts, was a graduate of Dartmouth College in Hanover, New Hampshire. He had lived in Missouri since 1843. A notable tribute was given him by the board of trustees of the Bowling Green Academy:

> *At a called meeting of the Board of Trustees of the Pike Academy, held in the town of Bowling Green, on the 29th of May, 1849, the following*

> *preamble and resolutions were presented by Mr. Porter to the Board, and, on motion unanimously adopted:*
>
> *WHEREAS, The Trustees of the Pike Academy at this place, since their last meeting, have received intelligence of the death of JOHN HUBBARD, Esq., the late Principal of the Institution, by Cholera, which occurred at the City of Jefferson, on the 15th inst., as a token of the respect with which we cherish his memory,*
>
> *Resolved, That we have received with deep regret, and an affected sorrow the sad news of the untimely end of our fellow-citizen and friend, John Hubbard; and especially are our sensibilities moved, when we reflect that he has fallen a victim to the fell destroyer far from home, kindred and friends, with none around him, save strangers, to perform "the last sad offices of humanity."*
>
> *Resolved, That we take pleasure in bearing testimony to the intellectual and moral worth of the deceased, and to the zeal, energy, and devotion with which he discharged the duties of his highly honorable and useful vocation, as an instructor of youth.*
>
> *Resolved, That in the death of Mr. Hubbard, the Academy in this place, of which he had charge for several years past, has lost an efficient and zealous teacher, and the community at large a useful and exemplary member.*
>
> *Resolved, That these resolutions be spread upon the records of the Board of Trustees, and that the Secretary of the Board furnish a copy of them to the editors of each of the newspapers of the county for publication, and also cause a copy of them to be forwarded to the aged parents of the deceased, who, we learn, reside in the town of Bremfield, in the State of Massachusetts.*[211]

His funeral was held in Bowling Green, Missouri, on June 14, 1849.[212] He was never married.

Captain Valentine (Val) Jordon (twenty-four) was the barkeeper on the *Monroe*. Val was from Louisville, Kentucky. He left a pregnant wife in that city; his only son was born less than a week after his death.

Benjamin Rush Lamb (twenty-eight) died on May 13, 1849.[213] He was the brother of Christiana Morris Lamb Hampton. He is mentioned in the Fair Hill Burial Ground in Philadelphia,[214] but I found no record of a tombstone for him there. His wife, Elizabeth Dubois Lamb, continued to Council Bluffs with their two children, John Isaac Lamb and Benjamin Rush Lamb Jr.

Elijah Malin (forty-one) of St. Louis. Elijah had been serving as a missionary for the Church of Jesus Christ of Latter-day Saints in Pennsylvania, primarily in Chester County. He completed his mission and joined with the Philadelphia company in Pittsburgh to travel back to his family in St. Louis. William Appleby had met Elijah previously, so Elijah was no stranger to the company. He was the first of the Philadelphia company to succumb to the cholera, in St. Louis, on May 5.

Edward McGlenry of Indiana died on the *Monroe* after leaving St. Louis. There is a newspaper report of a "Mr. Magtenerry" of Indiana dying. I believe this name is a misspelling of "McGlenry."

Fielding Rice McGrew (twenty-one) of Jeffersonville, Indiana. Some newspaper reports list his name as Rice Shirer. I believe they are the same person. When Rice was two years old, his father died. Two years later, his mother married John Daniel Shryer. Having been so young when his father died, and his mother remarrying, Fielding may have been known by both surnames. Rice died on the Sabbath morning, May 13, while being cared for in the "Presbyterian church."[215] I find it remarkable that his diary, along with his Scottish "dirk," made it back to Indiana and is still in possession of the family today. Most likely, his dirk, a long-thrusting dagger, was a family heirloom.

Mr. Meharey, the father of Charles Meharey of Baltimore, Maryland, was with the Jeffersonville company. In December 1876, Charles Meharey wrote a letter to at least two different newspapers in the Jeffersonville area looking for information about what happened to his father. His father is reported to have died of the cholera with Dr. Stephenson.[216]

Mr. Montgomery of Indiana.

Captain John P. Moore, ship's captain, died on May 12. He was a well-known steamboat commander from St. Louis. He had been a steamboat captain for at least seven years, so he was no stranger to the rivers. He had lived on Morgan Street, just a couple of blocks west of the Mississippi River, in the heart of downtown St. Louis.

Captain Moore's "colored boy."

J. Pincham of Indiana.

Joseph Ponto (about forty-five to forty-eight) of St. Charles, Missouri. He was one of the pilots on the *Monroe*. He died on May 9,[217] the day before the *Monroe* reached Jefferson City. Within a week of his death, his widow, Julia, filed his estate for probate in St. Charles County under the name of Joseph Panneton Sr. In both the 1850 Federal Census and the 1852 State Census for St. Charles County, Julia is listed as Julia Ponto. She is also listed as Julie Joseph Ponton when she remarried in 1856. Joseph is listed as Ponton when he married her in 1829. There is too much coincidence for this not to be the Joseph Ponto who was the pilot of the *Monroe*.

Jos. Rutherford, ship carpenter and watchman.

Preston F. Samuels (between twenty-nine and thirty-eight) of Shepherdsville, Kentucky, was left in St. Louis with two companions before the *Monroe* left port. On May 8,[218] he had been overcome with the cholera before the *Monroe* left port. It is assumed that he died there. Unfortunately, the names of his companions aren't known, nor is it known what happened to them. Preston was known as "the healthiest young [man] in the company, young and lively, he was a great favorite with his companions."[219] He had been an "Orderly Sergeant in Capt. B. R. Hardins' company of Ky. Infantry, in the Mexican war."[220] This would have been the Fourth Regiment of Kentucky Volunteers, received in October 1847 and disbanded in July 1848.

Dr. William Stephenson (fifty-nine), leader of the Jeffersonville company, died on May 10.

William Stephenson (between fourteen and sixteen), the son of Dr. Stephenson of the Jeffersonville company, died on May 13.

Mr. Williams, of Port Fulton, Indiana, died on May 8 or 9.[221] Today, Jeffersonville encompasses Port Fulton.

At least two **unknown Church members** from St. Louis.

The **ship's engineer** died on May 9.[222]

The **ship's second steward**.

Twelve boat hands.[223] I am not sure if any of the other members of the ship's crew are duplicated in this number. I would assume this number refers to the average ship laborer and not those who held positions such as engineer or fireman.

At least one of the ship's **mates**.[224]

Five unknown men who were "left in the old cabin"[225] with Lex (the only survivor). I have been unable to identify who they were, where they were going or where they originated from.

10
PERSONAL ACCOUNTS

One of the survivors gave a very heartfelt tribute to the citizens of Jefferson City when he wrote:

> *After the panic had somewhat subsided and the conduct of Carry became known, the generous citizens turned out to a man, all eager to assist, and attend the sick. They unweariedly watched night and day, and rendered every possible aid human generosity could suggest, burying the dead decently, and administering consolation to the survivors, and long will many of them be gratefully remembered—aye, life will close ere I forget the very humane and generous people of Jefferson City. The friends of the deceased will ever bless the stranger hands that soothed the last moments of the loved and lost; and the surviving ones, with their friends, will ever pray that the choices of Heaven's beneficent gifts be showered upon those benevolent citizens of Jefferson City. Words are all too cold, and passionless to describe the weight of gratitude I feel in my heart, or express the praise due those kind-hearted strangers; heaven alone can amply reward them, and to its care I commend them confidently.*[226]

Another one stated:

> *The sick, who were suddenly landed upon our shore, and who had no place to go at first, were very soon provided for by our citizens, and placed in our churches and vacant houses in different parts of the city. In many cases some*

> *of their friends and companions left them, but in every case the citizens of Jefferson provided for them without a thought of pecuniary consideration. Many citizens besides giving their personal attention to the sick and dying, and undergoing much fatigue and exposure, both day and night, paid money out of their own pockets, to assist in alleviating their condition, and rendering them comfortable; and all this without the expectation of fee or reward, except that of a feeling of consciousness of having discharged their duty toward their unfortunate fellow beings.*[227]

James E. McHenry remembered the following as a fourteen-year-old: "The people of Jefferson City then, as now, knew what to do in an emergency, and did it. When they learned the situation, they organized and took charge of the sick passengers, turned the churches, the court house and vacant houses into hospitals, and gave the sick and dying all the attention possible."[228]

Not all accounts had happy endings. One case tells of a

> *gentleman, his lady, and sister-in law, put up at one of our hotels. The same day, the lady was taken sick, and after lingering about three days died. The bed and bedding on which the lady died, was thrown away or destroyed. The husband of the lady saw this, and in paying his bill and the funeral expenses, paid for the bed, as we understand, without a murmur. We have been credibly informed that his whole bill at the hotel, including bed, coffin, shroud, Doctor's bill, and every other necessary expense, attending a burial did not amount to one half the amount listed by the Reveille.*[229]

E.S. Dils relates a fascinating account of his so-called escape from the clutches of death as he and Henry Bruner fled Jefferson City.

> *Henry Bruner and myself mounted swift horses, abandoned our wagons, baggage and clothing, and crossed the Missouri, leaving ill-fated Jefferson City to fight the plague as best it might. We rode fast and furious, a race with death, but he nearly caught us, for as we were trying to convince a farmer that we had not come from Jefferson City, I felt the first symptoms of the disease. During the night I vomited and drank laudanum* [a tincture made of 89 percent alcohol, 10 percent opium and 1 percent morphine] *by turns. Still I was determined to go on. It was the only thing to do, for the farmer would have put us out on the road anyhow. So we mounted again in the morning and rode on. I kept drinking my laudanum and it eased me. At Fulton, Mo., we bought a bottle of brandy and I drank*

> *it all; wanted to lie down under a tree and die, but Bruner whipped up my horse whenever I attempted to dismount, and thus we rode on. We passed the Jefferson City stage, with officers and men of the Monroe on board, fleeing for life, but they died before they reached St. Louis. On, on we rode all day, and the plague rode with us until dark; then we outstripped it and I began to revive.*
>
> *We rode on as fast as the horses would carry us, making the entire six hundred miles in twelve days.*[230]

We also have a newspaper account that praises the efforts of the local citizens and tells of the sadness of those they cared for:

> *Soon after the Monroe landed, the sick were removed, some to the Virginia Hotel, and others to various vacant houses in the city, where many of our citizens vied with each other in attentions to their wants. It pains us to say, that we have never witnessed such a fearful mortality, in any given number of cases, as has taken place since the arrival of this ill-fated steamer. All who have been attached with this "scourge of God," with comparatively few exceptions, have fallen victims. We have not been able to ascertain precisely the number of the dead.…Our Physicians have been active and constantly in attendance, and for their diligence and exposure, night and day deserve the public gratitude; but the malignant type of disease has thus far baffled medical skill in a large majority of the cases subjected to the treatment of our excellent Physicians. But three of the California Company alluded to now survive—some of them died before reaching this place—and the fatality has been little less alarming and terrible among the Mormon emigrants. The heart sickens at the contemplation of this awful dispensation of Providence—of whole families stricken down in a common grave, and of helpless little children, bereft of father and mother and cast upon the charities of the world—and all this desolation the result only a few hours! Heaven shower blessings on the heads of those who have generously stepped forward, not only to smoothe the pillow of the dying, and to bury the dead, but to console the bereft widow, and to feed and clothe, and have a mother's care for the little orphan.*[231]

A lady (one of the survivors, whose name is not listed) wrote a letter, published originally in the *Philadelphia North American* on May 24, 1849, that stated:

> *The people of Jefferson City behaved with great humility. An association of young men was formed to feed the sick. The Episcopal and Presbyterian churches, and an unoccupied hotel* [the "White House"] *were turned into hospitals, and the vacant houses in town placed at the disposition of the sick. In less than a week sixty of the passengers died, and in a short time thereafter twenty five of the generous citizens perished by the fell disease. The writer herself lost within three days her father, mother, brother and sister, and on the fourth day was herself attacked, but by diligent care recovered.*[232]

The *Jefferson Inquirer* also reported:

> *The citizens devoted themselves to the care of the sick, and, from that day to this, the unfortunate victims of the cholera have been nursed by day and night, by those who neglected their own business to attend to them. The citizens have done this cheerfully. They have provided, at their own expense, all the necessaries and even luxuries of the sick room. In this good work all classes have aided: laborers, mechanics, professional men, and the highest officers of State have vied with each other in supplying the wants of the sick, and in smoothing the pillow of the dying. All things have been provided in abundance, and much more offered than was needed. Few who were attacked have been saved, yet those who have owe their lives to the kindness of the citizens of this place. It is with the deepest regret that we have seen them so unjustly aspersed. Two weeks since we were not acquainted with a citizen of this place. Now, while life lasts a grateful memory will dwell upon may* [sic] *here with the deepest emotions. We can only attempt to express our gratitude, for we shall never be able to repay the obligations we are under to the citizens of Jefferson City.*[233]

Another female survivor wrote a letter, "To the Editors of the North American and U.S. Gazette," in which she stated:

> *Permit a woman who has been rescued from the very jaws of death by a people whom she never saw, and scarce ever heard of before the 16th* [10th] *of last month, the use of one of your columns for a single morning to express her gratitude, and to render honor to whom honor is due, as it is the only return she will ever be able to make for so much kindness, except to remember them in her prayers to the Almighty Ruler of the Heavens and the Earth. I ask this favor not because I have any right to demand it, but*

because the paper is an old acquaintance, my father having been a reader of it for a long series of years, whilst it was under the editorial supervision of Mr. Chandler.

I was a passenger on the steamer Monroe, bound from St. Louis to St. Joseph on the Missouri river, and on the morning of the 16th [10th] *of May, arrived at this port, the capital of the State. At the time of our arrival the dead, the dying and the sick were strewn every where about the ill-fated boat, and to get away from such a terrible pest house was the desire of every one. Before the boat touched the wharf the passengers were informed that it was impossible to continue the voyage on account of the cholera on board, and accordingly nearly two hundred of us, all carrying the seeds of the terrible pestilence in our systems, inundated this beautiful picturesque village. Not one human being in the town, so far as I know, had ever heard of one of us before, but to the honor of these people be it said that we were neither friendless or homeless.*

Immediately upon touching, our Captain deserted the boat, leaving the dead body of one of his own servants on board, shut himself up in a hotel, and forbid any access to him on any account. That night he left for St. Louis, and immediately after his arrival there, died of the epidemic. Oh! The sudden and terrible judgement. The clerk and owner of the Monroe ran away also, and through the columns of the Reveille, at St. Louis, calumniated most grossly a people whose kindness, sacrifices and philanthropy he was altogether unable to appreciate.

Being thus thrown ashore, our voyage broken up, and deserted by the officers of the boat, we were thrown, with the terrible pestilence among us, upon the charity of this village of about twelve hundred souls.

As might have been expected,—especially as the visitation of the cholera had been anticipated, and in such anticipation the village had been thoroughly cleansed, and was then perfectly healthy,—a great terror seized the people; but at the very threshold, in addition to the prompt energy of the physicians, appeared a guardian spirit—the Hon. James W. Morrow—whose self possession, cool courage, and indomitable energy, rallied around him a body of young men, without whose aid the sufferings of the sick and the dying must have forever remained untold. At his suggestion, the well were separated from the sick; the Episcopal and Presbyterian churches, and the White House and unoccupied hotel, were turned into hospitals, and the well furnished with all the vacant houses in the town.

And now the work of death commenced in right good earnest. In less than a week more than sixty of the Monroe's crew and passengers were in their graves, and at the end of about that time the dread scourge commenced its ravages amongst the citizens, and up to this date about twenty-five have died. In less than three days I saw father, mother, brother and sister, fall before the dread destroyer, and in the night of the fourth day my own summons came. I thought I had prepared to answer it, for I was without hope in this world, but Providence has ordered it otherwise, and I now live to tell the tale. To Dr. Wm. A. Davison, Judge Morrow, Capt. Parsons and Mr. Albert Baber I owe my life.

Never, never, shall I forget the horrors of the first night of my attack. It was dark and tempestuous, and I had just seen for the last time the purple corpses of my parents, brother and sister, but true to their great mission, the gentlemen I have named provided me with a female nurse, and some of them, I do not know who, watched in the adjoining room until the morning. Never shall I forget the remark of Judge Morrow immediately after I had passed, (although I did not then know it) the crisis of my disease. Coming in, he put his hand upon my forehead, felt my pulse and feet, and turning around spoke to Capt. Parsons, saying, "thank God, Parsons, she is saved." A re-action was taking place, and the next time I saw Dr. Davison, the kind, good man, he said to me; "you are out of danger if you are prudent."

The frequent recurrence of Judge Morrow's name in this incoherent sketch is excusable upon two grounds—he is not unknown to fame in the West as a jurist, and as a writer of politics and pungent humor; but the tribute is due to him as a philanthropist. The dangers to which he has exposed himself to render assistance to entire strangers, his activity and effective energy in a most appalling and trying crisis, his disinterested sacrifices, and his affectionate offices to the dead, make it his due. He seemed to be possessed of the power of ubiquity—being everywhere at the same time—when he was away, everything seemed to be out of joint—the sick called for him and invoked his assistance—even his tread upon the stair was the words of hope to me.

It was really affecting to see the rescued gather around him as he passed along the streets, and one morning when it was rumored that he had been assailed during the night by the fell destroyer, a thrill of horror ran through the whole town, and many of the city fathers flew to his residence to ascertain the truth. They returned almost shouting that it was nothing but a bilious attack brought on by exposure and fatigue.

I do not feel justified in closing this long—quite too long—epistle, without rendering in the name of the dead and living, to the people of Jefferson City, the Capital of the state of Missouri, my sincerest thanks—and most especially to Drs. Davison, Winston, Edwards, Dorris, Matthews and Krauser, to the Babers, Millers, Kerr, Hartt, Murray, Deitz, McKenzie, Cloney, Shubert, Green, the Parsons and Lusks, the Misses Lusk, and Mrs. Linn and her son, young Dr. Linn, and Dr. Wells, and others whose names I cannot now call to my memory.

May the Providence of God protect this town always.[234]

11
AFTERMATH

The year 1849 was one filled with many trials and challenges. It took a great deal of faith on the part of the passengers to embark on their various journeys. The first to leave their home and families was the company of members of the Church of Jesus Christ of Latter-day Saints from Philadelphia. Because of their faith in the Church, and at the urging of their prophet, Brigham Young, many were willing to forgo the pleasures of their current lives and risk everything to migrate to the Salt Lake Valley so they could gather with a larger population of Church members. Old and young, rich and poor, members from all walks of life had the faith to abandon their current status to make the long journey. Volumes have been written on the trials many suffered as they made their way across the unpopulated midsection of this country hoping to find a better life in the lands of the West.

Between the years 1847 and 1867, around 556,000 people made this long journey, many traveling from distant lands. St. Louis became a gathering place, as many foreigners sailed up the Mississippi, while others traveled down the Ohio River or cross country to reach the Missouri River. After making their way to places like Kanesville or Council Bluffs, Iowa, or even Winter Quarters, Nebraska, the "Saints" (as they became known) would travel by wagon train or handcart or just walk the one thousand miles plus to the Salt Lake Valley. This trek, weather permitting, would take an average of three months to complete.

The journey wasn't always easy. Not only were there wild animals to contend with, but also Indians were encountered in many places. Food was scarce, and shelter from the elements wasn't always readily available. The mortality rate was high. It is estimated that upward of 1,900 individuals died either on the way or shortly after their arrival in the Salt Lake Valley. Cholera and dysentery were the two most common illnesses.

As for the "gold-diggers" from Indiana, faith also had a lot to do with their journey. They too were leaving homes, families and jobs. The difference was that many anticipated returning, while the "Saints" looked on their migration as permanent. These forty-niners shared a similarity with the Argonauts from Greek mythology, with many even taking that name upon themselves. The Argonauts were heroes who took off on a quest to find the Golden Fleece. It was as if they were looking for a quick way to gain riches, just like the forty-niners did. One example of their faith is found in the words of the twenty-one-year-old Rice McGrew, who recorded the following in his diary: "Oh Lord prepare us all to meet the monstor [*sic*], for of a truth he comes like a thief in the night. May the dispensations of tThy [*sic*] Providence warn us all to make our peace with Thee, that we may all be prepared to go when ever Thy summond [*sic*] shall call us."[235]

Unfortunately, his diary entries appear to have stopped the next day, three to four days before he died.

Their journey followed much of the same path as the members of the Church took, up the Missouri River and across the plains. Some even traveled as far as Council Bluffs, Iowa, but the majority departed the Missouri River at places like Independence, Westport or St. Joseph, Missouri. Still others chose to travel by ship, crossing land at Panama, or traveled around Cape Horn. The Panama shortcut would take an average of two to three months, while the Cape Horn route took between four and eight months, at a much larger cost.

Traveling the three thousand miles across the plains from St. Joseph to California would take between three and seven months. Over thirty-two thousand gold-diggers traveled this route, with their wagons pulled by oxen or mules. They did not escape the diseases and trials the "Saints" had experienced. Not only did many of them die of cholera or diphtheria, but others also suffered from mountain fever and pneumonia.

Not everyone who reached their destination achieved the expectations they had hoped for. Some became disillusioned and struggled with their faith. Some wished they had never left their homelands and returned no richer in faith or monetary substance than when they left. Still others found what they were looking for. Many became rich, while others strengthened the faith they already had. I can't help but wonder: If we had to sacrifice and embark on a journey today such as those in this book had undertaken, would we have the perseverance to endure it well?

As William Clayton was fleeing Nauvoo in April 1846, he wrote the words to a hymn that provided strength to those facing the trials of their journey. His words apply to both companies as they journeyed. I hope we too can have faith like these travelers as we face the unknown trials of our day.

1. *Come, come, ye Saints, no toil nor labor fear;*
But with joy wend your way.
Though hard to you this journey may appear,
Grace shall be as your day.
'Tis better far for us to strive
Our useless cares from us to drive;
Do this, and joy your hearts will swell—
All is well! All is well!
2. *Why should we mourn or think our lot is hard?*
'Tis not so; all is right.
Why should we think to earn a great reward
If we now shun the fight?
Gird up your loins; fresh courage take.
Our God will never us forsake;
And soon we'll have this tale to tell—
All is well! All is well!
3. *We'll find the place which God for us prepared,*
Far away in the West,
Where none shall come to hurt or make afraid;
There the Saints will be blessed.
We'll make the air with music ring,
Shout praises to our God and King;
Above the rest these words we'll tell—
All is well! All is well!
4. *And should we die before our journey's through,*
Happy day! All is well!
We then are free from toil and sorrow, too;
With the just we shall dwell!
But if our lives are spared again
To see the Saints their rest obtain,
Oh, how we'll make this chorus swell—
All is well! All is well![236]

We also must not forget the citizens of Jefferson City. Their lives were disrupted as a swarm of people with the cholera landed on their shores. And what did they do? They did what any decent human being would do: they cared for them. Their behavior is a great tribute to the character of those who resided there.

On May 22, 2019, another disaster hit the borders of Jefferson City; an EF-3 tornado ripped a three-mile-long, one-mile-wide trail of destruction through the city. Fortunately, no immediate deaths were reported, and only a small amount of serious injuries were experienced. Once again, as happened in 1849, the citizens of Jefferson City stepped up and reached out to their neighbors to help clean up the city after the destruction. Again, we find that pride in a clean city was very much on the minds of the locals. In 1901, James McHenry remarked: "The people of Jefferson City then [1849], as now, knew what to do in an emergency, and did it. When they learned the situation they organized and took charge of the sick passengers....I presume there was not a man or woman in the town that did not do all in their power to relieve the sick and dying."[237]

One of the factors of the 2019 disaster was that, this time, people came from miles around to assist in the cleanup. This cleanup effort also included, ironically, the area members of the Church of Jesus Christ of Latter-day Saints—this time as survivors, not victims.

Appendix 1

SURVIVORS

Name	Company	Final Destination
Adams, Sarah Jane	Philadelphia	Returned to Philadelphia
Adams, Emma Elizabeth	Philadelphia	Returned to Philadelphia
Appleby, Augustin	Philadelphia	Salt Lake Valley
Appleby, Curles Shimm	Philadelphia	Salt Lake Valley
Appleby, Joseph Smith	Philadelphia	Salt Lake Valley
Appleby, Marth Ann	Philadelphia	Salt Lake Valley
*Appleby, Marinda Ann	Philadelphia	Salt Lake Valley
Appleby, Sarah Ann	Philadelphia	Salt Lake Valley
Appleby, Sarah Brown Price	Philadelphia	Salt Lake Valley
Appleby, William Ivins	Philadelphia	Salt Lake Valley
Appleby, William Price	Philadelphia	Salt Lake Valley
Austin, Brother	Philadelphia	Unknown
Beach, William Darrough	Jeffersonville	Returned to Jeffersonville
Bosley, George William	St. Louis	Salt Lake Valley
Bruner, Henry Clay	Jeffersonville	Returned to Jeffersonville
Dellinger, Henry Logan	Jeffersonville	California

Name	Company	Final Destination
Detty, Mr.	Jeffersonville	Unknown
Dils, Elias Safford	Jeffersonville	Returned to Jeffersonville
Eaby, Eliza Ann	Philadelphia	Salt Lake Valley
Eaby, John C.	Philadelphia	Salt Lake Valley
Edwards, Uriah	Jeffersonville	Returned to Jeffersonville
Farnham, Augustus	St. Louis	Salt Lake Valley
Farnham, Mary Jane	St. Louis	Salt Lake Valley
Farnham, Mary Jane Pottle	St. Louis	Salt Lake Valley
*Farnham, Ruth	St. Louis	Salt Lake Valley
Farnham, Sarah Mariah	St. Louis	Salt Lake Valley
Foster, Charles	Jeffersonville	Unknown
Franklin, Brother	Philadelphia	Unknown
Graham, Mr.	Jeffersonville	Unknown
Hammer, Joseph	Philadelphia	Unknown
Hampton, John William	Philadelphia	Returned to Philadelphia
Hampton, Benjamin Morgan	Philadelphia	Returned to Philadelphia
Hampton, Harriet L.	Philadelphia	Returned to Philadelphia
Hampton, John W., Jr.	Philadelphia	Returned to Philadelphia
Hampton, Mary Lamb	Philadelphia	Returned to Philadelphia
Hand, Elizabeth	Philadelphia	Traveled to Kanesville
Hand, William	Philadelphia	Traveled to Kanesville
Hodges, John D.	St. Louis	Returned to St. Louis
Kerr, J.W.	Jeffersonville	Unknown
King, John J.	Steamer crew	Unknown
Lafferty, William E.	Jeffersonville	California
Lamb, Elizabeth Dubois	Philadelphia	Salt Lake Valley
*Lamb, Elizabeth D.	Philadelphia	Salt Lake Valley
Lamb, Benjamin Rush, Jr.	Philadelphia	Salt Lake Valley

Name	Company	Final Destination
Lamb, John Isaac	Philadelphia	Salt Lake Valley
Lewis, Anne Elizabeth	St. Louis	Salt Lake Valley
*Lewis, Emily	St. Louis	Salt Lake Valley
Lewis, Emily Jennison Holman	St. Louis	Salt Lake Valley
Lewis, James Farrell	St. Louis	Salt Lake Valley
*Malin Council Bluffs	St. Louis	Salt Lake Valley
Malin, Margaret Ann	St. Louis	Salt Lake Valley
Malin, Mary Ann Bosley	St. Louis	Salt Lake Valley
Malin, James Elijah	St. Louis	Salt Lake Valley
Malin, John McGurkin	St. Louis	Salt Lake Valley
Malin, Samuel	St. Louis	Salt Lake Valley
Malin, Sarah	St. Louis	Salt Lake Valley
Murphy, James E.	Steamer crew	Returned to Indiana
Peters, F.W.	Steamer crew	Unknown
Pincham, R.M.	Jeffersonville	Unknown
Ruter, Rinaldo Robert	Jeffersonville	Returned to Jeffersonville
Sayers, Edward	St. Louis	Salt Lake Valley
Sayers, Ruth Daggett Vose	St. Louis	Salt Lake Valley
Ship's fireman	Steamer crew	Unknown
Smith, John Pearson	Philadelphia	Salt Lake Valley
Smith, George Opdycke	Philadelphia	Salt Lake Valley
Smith, Jane Hart Opdycke	Philadelphia	Salt Lake Valley
Smith, Mary Frances	Philadelphia	Salt Lake Valley
Smith, Theodore Augustus	Philadelphia	Salt Lake Valley
Wathen, James N.	Jeffersonville	Returned to Jeffersonville
Weathers, William	Jeffersonville	Returned to Jeffersonville
Williamson, Mr.	Jeffersonville	Unknown

Name	**Company**	**Final Destination**
Unknown couple	Philadelphia	Stayed behind to care for Elizabeth and William Hand
1 or 2 unknown couples	St. Louis or Philadelphia	Stayed behind in Jefferson City
2 unknown men	Jeffersonville	Stayed in St. Louis with Preston Samuels, fate unknown
Lex	Unknown	Joined the Union army in Davenport, Iowa

*Born after leaving Jefferson City

Appendix 2
KNOWN DEATHS

Name	Company	Burial Place
Adams, Elizabeth	Philadelphia	Jefferson City
Adams, Hester Ann	Philadelphia	Jefferson City
Adams, William D.	Philadelphia	Jefferson City
Bachelor, Sister	Philadelphia	Jefferson City
Baily, Robert	unknown	Jefferson City
Beach, William	Jeffersonville	Jefferson City
Brown, Sister	St. Louis	Jefferson City
Chaflin, Mr.	Jeffersonville?	Missouri River?
Darrough, James	Jeffersonville	Jefferson City
Davenport, J.	Jeffersonville	Jefferson City
Donsed, Mr.	Jeffersonville	Jefferson City
Eaby, Eliza Pierce	Philadelphia	Jefferson City
Eaby, Eliza Pierce, child	Philadelphia	Jefferson City
Edgerton, Mr.	Jeffersonville	Jefferson City
Edgington, John	Jeffersonville	Jefferson City
Edgington, William	Jeffersonville	Jefferson City
Edmonston, John	Jeffersonville	Jefferson City

Name	Company	Burial Place
Granger, Sabra	St. Louis	Jefferson City
Hall (gender unknown)	Philadelphia	Jefferson City
Hammer, Sister (Mary?)	Philadelphia	Jefferson City
Hammer, Sister, child	Philadelphia	Jefferson City
Hampton, Christiana Morris Lamb	Philadelphia	Jefferson City
Hampton, Isaac Lamb	Philadelphia	Jefferson City
Hand, Elizabeth Ann Merrill	Philadelphia	Jefferson City
Hand, William	Philadelphia	Jefferson City
Hodges, Lavina Price	St. Louis	Jefferson City
Hubbard, John	Bowling Green, Missouri	Jefferson City
Jordon, Captain Val	steamer crew	Jefferson City
Lamb, Benjamin Rush	Philadelphia	Jefferson City
Malin, Elijah	Philadelphia	St. Louis
McGlenry, Edward	Jeffersonville	Missouri River
McGrew, Rice	Jeffersonville	Jefferson City
Meharey, Mr.	Jeffersonville	Jefferson City
Montgomery, Mr.	Jeffersonville	Jefferson City
Moore, Captain John P.	steamer crew	St. Louis
Moore, Captain John P. ("colored boy")	steamer crew	Jefferson City
Pincham, J.	Jeffersonville	Jefferson City
Ponto, Joseph	steamer crew	Jefferson City
Rutherford, Jos.	steamer crew	Jefferson City
Samuels, Preston	Jeffersonville	St. Louis
Ship's second steward	steamer crew	Jefferson City
Ship's engineer	steamer crew	Jefferson City
Ship's mate	steamer crew	Jefferson City

Name	Company	Burial Place
Ship's mate	steamer crew	Jefferson City
Smith, Charles	Philadelphia	Jefferson City
Stephenson, Dr. William	Jeffersonville	Jefferson City
Stephenson, William	Jeffersonville	Jefferson City
Unknown brother	St. Louis	Missouri River
Unknown brother	St. Louis	Jefferson City
Williams, Mr.	Jeffersonville	Missouri River
Twelve boat hands	steamer crew	Jefferson City
Five unknown men	unknown	Jefferson City

NOTES

Introduction

1. Farmer and Woods, "Sanctuary on the Mississippi," 47.
2. "Ship of Death," *Weekly Herald*. This page of the newspaper is misprinted with the incorrect date of October 16, 1892.

Chapter 1

3. Crawley, *Descriptive Bibliography of the Mormon Church*, 358.
4. Appleby, "William I. Appleby autobiography and journal, 1848–1856."
5. Ibid., 250.
6. Woodruff, letter, Cambridge, Massachusetts, to Alexander Badlam, 3.
7. Webster, *American Dictionary of the English Language*.
8. "Proclamation of The Twelve Apostles of The Church of Jesus Christ, of Latter Day Saints." April 6, 1845.
9. "Proclamation of the Twelve Apostles of The Church of Jesus Christ of Latter-day Saints (April 6 and October 22, 1845)."
10. Gillespie, "Steamboat Design & Operations," in *Wild River, Wooden Boats*, 27.
11. Appleby, "William I. Appleby autobiography and journal, 1848–1856," 253–54.
12. "Mormon Method of Treating Cholera." *Palmyra Missouri Whig*.

13. Appleby, "William I. Appleby autobiography and journal, 1848–1856," 254.
14. Ibid.
15. Appleby, "Br. O. Hyde."
16. "Helpful Hints for Steamboat Passengers," Malcolm Price Laboratory School.
17. Martin, "Liverpool to New Orleans 6 Feb 1849–18 Apr 1849," *Saints By Sea*.
18. Turner, *Voices of Missouri's Rivers*, 236.
19. Diary of Rice McGrew.
20. "The Mormons," *Ripley Bee*.

Chapter 2

21. "Old Time Travellers," *Jeffersonville News*.
22. "Over the Plains in '49 Was No Pleasant Journey," *Jeffersonville National Democrat*.
23. "Gold Diggings—Jeffersonville California Company—Dr. Stephenson," *Cincinnati Western Christian Advocate*.
24. "Over the Plains in '49."
25. Jones, "Life on the Miners' Frontier," *Daily Life on the 19th Century American Frontier*, 123.
26. "Gold Diggings."
27. Diary of Rice McGrew.
28. "Friend Curtiss," *Evening Post*.
29. "Ship of Death," *Jeffersonville News*.
30. "Friend Curtiss."
31. Diary of Rice McGrew.
32. "Ship of Death," *Jeffersonville News*.
33. *Illinois Daily Journal*, May 16, 1849.

Chapter 3

34. Way, *Way's Packet Directory, 1848–1983*, 329.
35. "From the Metropolitan of the 15th, Cholera in Jefferson City," *Frontier Guardian*.
36. "Steamer Monroe," *Daily New Albany Democrat*.
37. Cordell Jr. "Letter to his father."
38. Woodruff, letter, Cambridge, Massachusetts, to Alexander Badlam, 3.

39. Brasseaux and Fontenot, *Steamboats on Louisiana's Bayous*, 215.
40. *Daily Evansville Journal*, April 7, 1854.
41. "Loss of the Monroe," *Louisville Daily Courier*.

Chapter 4

42. Giffen, *Walks in Water*, 120.
43. "Cholera West," *Boston Semi-Weekly Atlas*.
44. "Friend Curtiss," *Evening Post*.
45. Holliday and Swain, "A Migration of Strangers," in *World Rushed In*, 77.
46. *World Rushed In*, note 77, 469.
47. "Old Days on the Missouri" *Saint Paul Globe*.
48. "Upper Missouri Trade Opening for St. Louis," *St. Louis Globe-Democrat*, September 30, 1906.
49. "Terrible Mortality," *Daily New Albany Democrat*.
50. "Californians at Independence," *Richmond Whig and Public Advertiser*. This paper was also known as *Richmond Daily Whig* and *Richmond Semi-Weekly Whig*. This page is incorrectly printed as May 28, 1849.
51. "Cholera," *Jefferson Inquirer*.
52. "Ship of Death," *Jeffersonville News*.
53. "Terrible Mortality."
54. Clark, *Gold Rush Diary*, 2–3.
55. "Ship of Death."
56. "Over the Plains in '49 Was No Pleasant Journey," *Jeffersonville National Democrat*.
57. "Ship of Death," *Weekly Herald*. This page of the newspaper is misprinted with the incorrect date of October 16, 1892.
58. *Melchisedek and Aaronic Herald*.
59. Holliday and Swain, "A Migration of Strangers," in *World Rushed In*, 76.
60. "Mortality on Mississippi Steamboats," *Cleveland Herald*.
61. Holliday and Swain, *World Rushed In*, 76.
62. Lepley, *Packets to Paradise*, 82.

Chapter 5

63. "Mortality on Mississippi Steamboats," *Cleveland Herald*, quoting an article in the *Louisville Journal* (date unknown).

64. Diary of Rice McGrew.
65. Appleby, "William I. Appleby autobiography and journal, 1848–1856," 254.
66. "Ship of Death," *Jeffersonville News*.
67. Diary of Rice McGrew.
68. "Ship of Death," *Jeffersonville News*.
69. "Gold Diggings—Jeffersonville California Company—Dr. Stephenson," *Cincinnati Western Christian Advocate*.
70. Decker and Giffen, "The Land of Sun Down," in *Diaries of Peter Decker*, 51.
71. Clark, *Gold Rush Diary*, 2.
72. Read and Gaines, "Volume 1: Washing City to Bruff's Camp," *Gold Rush*, 5.
73. Appleby, "William I. Appleby autobiography and journal, 1848–1856," 198.
74. Ibid., 255.
75. "Cholera," *Jefferson Inquirer*.
76. "Ship of Death," *Jeffersonville News*.
77. "Gold Diggings—Jeffersonville California Company—Dr. Stephenson," *Cincinnati Western Christian Advocate*.
78. "Abandoned," *Louisiana Banner*.
79. "Journey Westward Was Cut Short by Cholera," *Jeffersonville Evening News*.
80. "Cholera," *Jefferson Inquirer*.
81. Hattervig, "Jefferson Landing," 286.
82. Gordon, "Fearful Visitation," In *Fire, Pestilence, and Death*, 54.
83. "Plague," *Jefferson City Daily Press*.
84. Hattervig, "Jefferson Landing," 286.
85. Ibid., 286.
86. "Steamer Monroe," *Jefferson Inquirer*.
87. "Messrs. Editors," *Jefferson Inquirer*.
88. "Missouri House," *Jeffersonian Republican*.
89. "Steamer Monroe," *New Albany Democrat Daily Courier*.
90. "Local Matters," *Daily Morning Post*.
91. "Steamer Monroe," *Jefferson Inquirer*.
92. "Further Particulars," *Indiana Palladium*.
93. "Centennial Fourth," *State Journal*.
94. "Ferries," Laws of the State of Missouri, 1841, 168–69.
95. "Ferries," Laws of the State of Missouri, 1838, 214–16.
96. "Centennial Fourth."

97. "Jefferson City Steam Ferry Boat," *Saturday Morning Visitor.*
98. "Cholera," *Jefferson Inquirer.*
99. "Golden Era of River Recalled By Barge Line," *Jefferson City* (MO) *Sunday News and Tribune*, March 31, 1935.
100. Lass, "The Expanding Frontier," in *Navigating the Missouri*, 153.
101. "Cholera," *Jefferson Inquirer.*
102. Larkin, "Missouri Heritage," *Kansas City Star.*
103. Montgomery, "Mexican War, Gold Rush, Train Wrecks in Life of G. Bickerton Winston," *Sunday News and Tribune.*
104. Giffen, *Walks in Water*, 120.
105. "Cholera," *Jefferson Inquirer.*
106. Ibid.
107. "A Few Plain Facts Relative to the Ill Fated Steamer Monroe," *Daily New Albany Democrat.*
108. "Gold Diggings—Jeffersonville California Company—Dr. Stephenson," *Cincinnati Western Christian Advocate.*
109. "White House," *Daily Argus.*
110. "Fire, and Remarkable Preservation of Property," *Jeffersonian Republican*, January 22, 1842.
111. Gordon, "Fearful Visitation," in *Fire, Pestilence, and Death*, 50–51.
112. Cordell Jr., "Letter to his father."
113. "Friend Curtiss," *Evening Post.*
114. Appleby, "William I. Appleby autobiography and journal, 1848–1856," 256.
115. "Cholera in the West." *North American and United States Gazette.*
116. "Death of Dr. John H. Edwards," *Peoples Tribune.*
117. "In Memorium," *Peoples Tribune.*
118. "Death of Dr. Abbot," *Fulton Telegraph.*
119. "Friend Curtiss," *Evening Post.*
120. "Journey Westward Was Cut Short by Cholera," *Jeffersonville Evening News* (originally cited in *Jeffersonville (IN) Evening News*, January 19, 1904).
121. Ibid.
122. "Shinplasters," Past & Present.
123. "Messrs. Editors."
124. Cordell Jr., "Letter to his father."
125. "Steamer Monroe," *Inquirer.*
126. "Messrs. Editors."
127. Clark, *Gold Rush Diary*, 2–3.
128. Sayers, *Jefferson Inquirer.*

129. *History of the Ohio Falls Cities and Their Counties*, 440.
130. "Terrible Mortality," *Daily New Albany Democrat*.
131. Appleby, "William I. Appleby autobiography and journal, 1848–1856," 256.
132. Appleby, "For the Frontier Guardian," *Frontier Guardian*.
133. "Missouri Heritage," *Kansas City Star*.
134. "Last-Ditch Effort to Save Lohman's Landing Launched," *Jefferson City Post-Tribune*.
135. "Cholera," *Jefferson Inquirer*.
136. Farmer and Woods, "Sanctuary on the Mississippi," 49. From a Nathaniel Felt family historian, originally quoted in Kate B. Carter, *Our Pioneer Heritage* (Salt Lake City, UT: Daughters of Utah Pioneers, 1959), 5: 445–46.
137. "History of Jefferson City Outlined for Cole County Historical Society," *Sunday News and Tribune*.
138. "Gold Diggings—Jeffersonville California Company—Dr. Stephenson," *Cincinnati Western Christian Advocate*.
139. Chappell, *History of the Missouri River*, 92.
140. "Journey Westward Was Cut Short by Cholera."
141. *Missouri Courier*, May 24, 1849.
142. "Cholera Cases," *North American and United States Gazette*.
143. "Laid Up," *Glasgow Weekly Times*.
144. "History of Cole County," in *History of Cole, Moniteau, Morgan, Benton, Miller, Maries and Osage Counties Missouri*, 283.
145. "Terrible Mortality," *Daily New Albany Democrat*.
146. McHenry, "Document bearing the signature of James Edgar McHenry."
147. City of Jefferson. Council Minutes, 1849–1850, 238.
148. Ibid., 239.
149. Loren Humphrey, "Evils of Cities and Medical School Problems," in *Quinine and Quarantine Missouri Medicine through the Years* (Columbia: University of Missouri Press, 2000), 41.

Chapter 6

150. Cooperman, "Take Care, and Don't Take the Cholera," *St. Louis Magazine*.
151. "Treatment of Cholera," *Glasgow Times*.
152. Giffen, *Walks in Water*, 121.

153. Baker, "Illness and Mortality in Nineteenth-Century Mormon Immigration," 86.
154. "Cholera in the West," *New York Weekly Herald*.
155. "Cholera," Audio English.
156. Smyser, "Dr. Smyser's Report," *Republican Banner*.
157. Godwin, "Saint Louis Cholera Epidemic of 1849," 12.
158. Ibid., 13.
159. "Plague," *Jefferson City Daily Press*.
160. "Cholera," *Jefferson Inquirer*.
161. Ibid.
162. Holliday and Swain, "Fitting for a Start," in *World Rushed In*, 89.
163. "Friend Curtiss," *Evening Post*.
164. Turner, *Voices of Missouri's Rivers*, 236–37.
165. "Helpful Hints for Steamboat Passengers," Malcolm Price Laboratory School.
166. "Mortality on Mississippi Steamboats," *Cleveland Herald*.
167. "Mr. Editor," *Boston Weekly Messenger*.
168. "Cholera," *Columbia Missouri Statesman*.
169. "Cholera," *Jefferson City Inquirer*.
170. Holliday and Swain, "A Migration of Strangers," in *World Rushed In*, 77.
171. "Cholera," *Jefferson Inquirer*.
172. "Cholera on a Western Steamboat," *New Orleans Daily Crescent*.
173. "The Plague," *Jefferson City Daily Press*.
174. Jones, Journal of the House.

Chapter 7

175. "Friend Curtiss," *Evening Post*.
176. Appleby, "Br. O. Hyde," *Frontier Guardian*.
177. "Historical Department journal history of the Church, 1896–2001 July; 1840–1849; 1849 January–July."
178. Appleby, "Br. O. Hyde."
179. Emma S. Woodruff collection, 1832–1919.

Chapter 8

180. "Deaths of a Family," *Woodstock Mercury, and Windsor County Advertiser*.

181. Ward, "Philadelphia Branch Membership, 1840–1854."
182. "Historical Society of Pennsylvania, Deaths & Burials," Find My Past.
183. "Sonoma District Pioneers," *Sonoma Democrat.*
184. Emma S. Woodruff collection, 1832–1919.
185. *Louisville Daily Courier*, May 21, 1849.
186. *Jefferson Inquirer*, September 15, 1849.
187. Emma S. Woodruff collection, 1832–1919.
188. "Messrs. Editors," *Jefferson Inquirer.*
189. "Plague," *Jefferson City Daily Press.*
190. "Utah Deaths and Burials, 1888–1946," Family Search.
191. "Plague," *Jefferson City Daily Press.*
192. Emma S. Woodruff collection, 1832–1919.
193. "Army Correspondence," *Daily Gazette.*

Chapter 9

194. Ward, "Philadelphia Branch Membership, 1840–1854."
195. "Sad Mortality," *Lancaster Gazette.*
196. "Historical Society of Pennsylvania, Deaths & Burials," Find My Past.
197. Ibid.
198. Appleby, "William I. Appleby autobiography and journal, 1848–1856," 255.
199. Cole County, Missouri, probate case files, estate #37-A, W.D. Adams (1849) Probate Court, Jefferson City, Missouri. The name of Bailey is a best guess of what the handwriting is saying.
200. McMullen, "Hamer Robinson McMullen Families," family Bible belonging to Samuel and Mary Ann Bosley.
201. "Turned Back," *Ohio Observer.*
202. Ibid.
203. Woodruff, Journals and papers, 1828–1898; Wilford Woodruff Journals, 1833–1898; Wilford Woodruff Journal, 1847 January–1853 December; Church History Library.
204. Emma S. Woodruff collection, 1832–1919.
205. Woodruff, Journals.
206. Philadelphia Branch Membership, Mormon Historic Sites.
207. "Died," *Philadelphia Inquirer and National Gazette.*
208. Find A Grave, memorial page for Christiana Morris Lamb Hampton (1816–May 10, 1849).

209. Find A Grave, memorial page for Isaac Hampton (1846–May 11, 1849).
210. Ancestry.com. Massachusetts, Town and Vital Records, 1620-1988 [database on-line]. Provo, UT, USA: Ancestry.com Operations, Inc., 2011.
211. "Tribute of Respect," *Democratic Banner*.
212. "Masonic Procession," *Democratic Banner*.
213. "Died," *Philadelphia Inquirer and National Gazette*.
214. Find A Grave, memorial page for Benjamin Rush Lamb (August 23, 1821–May 13, 1849).
215. "Gold Diggings—Jeffersonville California Company—Dr. Stephenson," *Cincinnati Western Christian Advocate*.
216. "Information Wanted," *Jeffersonville Evening News*.
217. Appleby, "William I. Appleby autobiography and journal, 1848–1856," 254.
218. Diary of Rice McGrew.
219. Ibid.
220. *Louisville Daily Courier*, May 23, 1849.
221. "Ship of Death," *Jeffersonville News*.
222. Appleby, autobiography and journal, 254.
223. Woodruff letter, Cambridgeport, Massachusetts, to Alexander Badlam.
224. Wilford Woodruff letter.
225. "Army Correspondence," *Daily Gazette*.

Chapter 10

226. "A Few Plain Facts Relative to the Ill-Fated Steamer Monroe," *Daily New Albany Democrat*.
227. "Steamer Monroe," *Jefferson Inquirer*.
228. "Plague," *Jefferson City Daily Press*.
229. "Steamer Monroe," *Jefferson Inquirer*.
230. "Ship of Death," *Weekly Herald*.
231. "From the Metropolitan of the 15th, Cholera in Jefferson City," *Frontier Guardian*.
232. "Cholera on a Western Steamboat," *New Orleans Daily Crescent*.
233. "Messrs. Editors," *Jefferson Inquirer* (Jefferson City, MO), May 26, 1849.
234. "To the Editors of the North American and U.S. Gazette," *North American and United States Gazette* (Philadelphia), July 7, 1849, http://0-find.galegroup.com.iii.slcl.org/ncnp/.

Chapter 11

235. Diary of Rice McGrew.
236. "Come, Come, Ye Saints," *Hymns of The Church of Jesus Christ of Latter-day Saints*, 30.
237. "Plague," *Jefferson City Daily Press*.

BIBLIOGRAPHY

Online Newspaper Sources Consulted

ChroniclingAmerica.loc.gov

GenealogyBank.com

Newspapers.com

St. Louis County Library

Books and Articles

Appleby, W.I. "Br. O. Hyde." *Frontier Guardian*, July 25, 1849.

———. "For the Frontier Guardian." *Frontier Guardian* (Kanesville, IA), June 27, 1849. https://archive.org.

——— "William I. Appleby autobiography and journal, 1848–1856." Accessed February 1, 2019. https://catalog.churchofjesuschrist.org.

Audio English. "Cholera." https://www.audioenglish.org.

Baker, Shane A. "Illness and Mortality in Nineteenth-Century Mormon Immigration." *Mormon Historical Studies* 2 no. 2 (2001): 86. http://mormonhistoricsites.org.

Boston (MA) Semi-Weekly Atlas. "The Cholera West." May 23, 1849.

Boston Weekly Messenger. "Mr. Editor." May 30, 1849.

Brasseaux, Carl A., and Keith P. Fontenot. *Steamboats On Louisiana's Bayous: A History and Directory.* Baton Rouge: Louisiana State University Press. 2004.

Chappell, Phil E. *A History of the Missouri River.* Topeka, KS: State Print Office, 1906.

Cincinnati Western Christian Advocate. "Gold Diggings—Jeffersonville California Company—Dr. Stephenson." July 4, 1849.

City of Jefferson. City Clerk. Council Minutes. 1849–1850, 238. http://documents.jeffcitymo.org.

Clark, Thomas D. *Gold Rush Diary Being the Journal of Elisha Douglas Perkins on the Overland Trail in the Spring and Summer of 1849*. Lexington: University Press of Kentucky, 2015.

Cleveland (OH) Herald. "Mortality on Mississippi Steamboats." May 25, 1849.

Columbia Missouri Statesman. "Cholera." April 27, 1849.

Cooperman Jeannette. "Take Care, and Don't Take the Cholera." *St. Louis Magazine*. June 25, 2010. https://www.stlmag.com.

Cordell, Presley, Jr. "Letter to his father." 1849. On file at the Cole County Historical Society. Jefferson City, Missouri.

Crawley, Peter. *A Descriptive Bibliography of the Mormon Church, Volume One, 1830–1847*. Provo, UT: Religious Studies Center, Brigham Young University. 1997.

Daily Argus (St. Louis, MO). "White House." August 28, 1840.

Daily Evansville (IN) Journal, April 7, 1854.

Daily Gazette (Davenport, IA). "Army Correspondence." December 23, 1861.

Daily Morning Post (Pittsburgh, PA). "Local Matters." May 1, 1849.

Daily New Albany (IN) Democrat. "A Few Plain Facts Relative to the Ill Fated Steamer Monroe." June 25, 1849.

———. "The Steamer Monroe." May 21, 1849.

———. "Terrible Mortality." May 18, 1849.

Daily Picayune (New Orleans, LA). "Loss of Steamer Monroe." March 29, 1854.

Decker, Peter, and Helen S. Giffen. *The Diaries of Peter Decker: Overland to California in 1849 and Life in the Mines, 1850–1851.* Georgetown, CA: Talisman Press, 1966.

Democratic Banner (Louisiana MO). "Masonic Procession." June 11, 1849.

———. "Tribute of Respect." June 4, 1849.

Diary of Rice McGrew, transcribed by Marc L. Liston, in possession of Nina L. Steiner, "Rose/McGrew/Turner/Klaenhammer Family" (genealogy) by Fred Rose, compiler (2008); published on the internet by the RootsWeb WorldConnect Project, https://wc.rootsweb.com.

Erwin, Vicki Berger, and James Erwin. *Steamboat Disasters of the Lower Missouri River.* Charleston, SC: The History Press, 2020.

Evening Post (New York). "Friend Curtiss." June 20, 1849.

Farmer, Thomas L., and Fred E. Woods. "Sanctuary on the Mississippi: St. Louis as Way Station for Mormon Emigration." *The Confluence* 9, no. 2 (2018): 42–56. https://www.lindenwood.edu.

"Ferries." Laws of the State of Missouri, Passed at the First Session of the Ninth General Assembly, begun and held at the city of Jefferson: Printed by order of the Secretary of State, by Chambers & Knapp-Republican Office, 1841, 168–69.

"Ferries." Laws of the State of Missouri, Passed at the First Session of the Tenth General Assembly, begun and held at the city of Jefferson: Printed by order of the Secretary of State, by Chambers & Knapp-Republican Office, 1838, 214–16.

Find A Grave. Memorial page for Isaac Hampton (1846–May 11, 1849), Find A Grave Memorial no. 200166747, citing Fair Hill Burial Ground, Philadelphia, Philadelphia County, Pennsylvania, USA; Maintained by SusanG (contributor 47958392). Accessed July 26, 2019. https://www.findagrave.com.

———. Memorial page for Benjamin Rush Lamb (August 23, 1821–May 13, 1849), Find A Grave Memorial no. 200683499, citing Fair Hill Burial Ground, Philadelphia, Philadelphia County, Pennsylvania, USA; Maintained by SusanG (contributor 47958392). Accessed July 26, 2019. https://www.findagrave.com.

———. Memorial page for Christiana Morris Lamb Hampton (1816–May 10, 1849), Find A Grave Memorial no. 143211794, citing Fair Hill Burial Ground, Philadelphia, Philadelphia County, Pennsylvania, USA; Maintained by SusanG (contributor 47958392). https://www.findagrave.com.

Frontier Guardian (Kanesville, IA). "From the Metropolitan of the 15th, Cholera in Jefferson City." June 13, 1849. https://archive.org.

Fulton (MO) Telegraph. "Death of Dr. Abbot." January 24, 1873.

Giffen, Lawrence Everett. *Walks In Water: The Impact of Steamboating on the Lower Missouri River.* Jefferson City, MO: Giffen Enterprises, 2001.

Gillespie, Michael. *Wild River, Wooden Boats: True Stories of Steamboating on the Missouri River.* Stoddard, WI: Heritage Press, 2000.

Glasgow (MO) Times. "Treatment of Cholera." May 24, 1849.

Glasgow (MO) Weekly Times. "Laid Up." May 17, 1849.

Godwin, Bette. "The Saint Louis Cholera Epidemic of 1849 as It Appeared in the Newspapers." Master's thesis, St. Louis University, 1951.

Gordon, Christopher Alan. *Fire, Pestilence, and Death: St. Louis 1849.* St. Louis: Missouri History Museum Press. 2018.

Hattervig, Eldon. "Jefferson Landing: A Commercial Center of the Steamboat Era." *Missouri Historical Review* 74, no. 3 (1980): 277–99. https://digital.shsmo.org.

"Helpful Hints for Steamboat Passengers." Malcom Price Laboratory School, University of Northern Iowa. https://iowahist.uni.edu.

"Historical Department Journal History of the Church, 1830–2008; 1840–1849; 1849 January–July." Church History Library. Accessed July 8, 2019. https://catalog.churchofjesuschrist.org.

"Historical Society of Pennsylvania, Deaths & Burials." 2019. Find My Past. https://www.findmypast.com.

"History of Cole County." In *The History of Cole, Moniteau, Morgan, Benton, Miller, Maries and Osage Counties, Missouri*, 203–309. Easley, SC: Southern Historial Press, 1978.

History of the Ohio Falls Cities and Their Counties. Cleveland, OH: L.A. Williams, 1882.

Holliday, J.S., and William Swain. *The World Rushed In: The California Gold Rush Experience*. New York: Simon & Schuster, 1981.

Hymns of The Church of Jesus Christ of Latter-day Saints. Salt Lake City: Church of Jesus Christ of Latter-day Saints, 1985.

Illinois Daily Journal (Springfield, IL), May 16, 1849.

Indiana Palladium (Vevay, IN). "Further Particulars." May 26, 1849.

Jefferson City (MO) Daily Press. "The Plague." March 17, 1901.

Jefferson City (MO) Post-Tribune. "Last-Ditch Effort to Save Lohman's Landing Launched." February 10, 1969.

Jefferson City (MO) Sunday News and Tribune. "Golden Era of River Recalled by Barge Line." March 31, 1935.

Jeffersonian Republican (Jefferson City, MO). "Fire, and Remarkable Preservation of Property." January 22, 1842.

———. "Missouri House." April 10, 1841.

Jefferson Inquirer (Jefferson City, MO), September 15, 1849.

———. "Cholera." May 5, 1849.

———. "Cholera." May 12, 1849.

———. "Cholera." May 19, 1849.

———. "Messrs. Editors." May 26, 1849.

———. "The Steamer Monroe." May 19, 1849.

Jeffersonville (IN) Evening News. "Information Wanted." December 11, 1876.

———. "Journey Westward Was Cut Short by Cholera." January 19, 1904.

———. "Journey Westward Was Cut Short by Cholera." January 25, 1954.

Jeffersonville (IN) National Democrat. "Over the Plains in '49 Was No Pleasant Journey." August 27, 1897.

Jeffersonville (IN) News. "Old Time Travellers." May 3, 1892.

———. "The Ship of Death." September 17, 1892.

Jones, Mary Ellen. *Daily Life on the 19th Century American Frontier.* Westport, CT: Greenwood Press, 1998.

Journal of the House, Sixteenth General Assembly, First Session, 1851, Appendix and Index, pages 184 and 187, General Assembly, Record Group 550, Missouri State Archives, Jefferson City, Missouri, https://www.sos.mo.gov/mdh.

Lancaster (OH) Gazette. "Sad Mortality." June 1, 1849. https://chroniclingamerica.loc.gov.

Larkin, Lew. "Missouri Heritage." *Kansas City (MO) Star*. December 28, 1968.

Lass, William E. *Navigating The Missouri: Steamboating on Nature's Highway, 1819–1935*. Norman, OK: Arthur H. Clark, 2008.

Lepley, John G. *Packets to Paradise: Steamboating to Fort Benton*. Missoula, MT: Pictorial Histories Publishing, 2001.

Liston, Marc. "Rose/McGrew/Turner/Klaenhammer Family." Roots Web World Connect Project. 2001. https://wc.rootsweb.com.

Louisiana (MO) Banner. "Abandoned." May 21, 1849.

Louisville (KY) Daily Courier. May 21, 1849.

———. May 23, 1849.

———. "The Loss of the Monroe." April 8, 1854.

Martin, John. Autobiography. "Liverpool to New Orleans 6 Feb 1849–18 Apr 1849." *Saints By Sea: Latter-day Saint Immigration to America*. Provo, UT: Brigham Young University. 2000. https://mormonmigration.lib.byu.edu.

"Massachusetts, Town and Vital Records, 1620–1988" Database online. Provo, UT: Ancestry.com Operations Inc., 2011.

McHenry, James Edgar. Jefferson City, MO. 1893. "Document bearing the signature of James Edgar McHenry." On the letterhead of the office of the City Clerk of Jefferson City, Missouri. On file at the Cole County Historical Society, Jefferson City, Missouri.

McMullen, John. "Hammer Robinson McMullen Families." Roots Web World Connect Project. 2014. https://wc.rootsweb.com.

———. "Hamer Robinson McMullen Families." Family Bible belonging to Samuel and Mary Ann Bosley. Updated January 26, 2014. Published online by the RootsWeb WorldConnect Project. https://wc.rootsweb.com.

Melchisedek and Aaronic Herald (Covington, KY), June 1849. Internet Archive. https://archive.org.

Missouri Courier (Hannibal), May 24, 1849.

"Missouri Probate Case Files." 1849. *Estate* #37-A. W.D. Adams. Probate Court. Cole County, Jefferson City, Missouri, probate case files, estate.

Montgomery, Helen Clark. "Mexican War, Gold Rush, Train Wrecks in Life of G. Bickerton Winston." *Sunday News and Tribune (Jefferson City)*, May 6, 1945.

New Albany (IN) Democrat Daily Courier. "The Steamer Monroe." May 24, 1849.

New Orleans (LA) Daily Crescent. "Cholera on a Western Steamboat." July 16, 1849.

New York Weekly Herald. "Cholera in the West." May 26, 1849.

North American and United States Gazette (Philadelphia). "Cholera Cases." June 1, 1849.

———. "Cholera in the West." May 28, 1849.

———. "To the Editors of the North American and U.S. Gazette." July 7, 1849.

Ohio Observer (Hudson OH). "Turned Back." June 20, 1849.

Palmyra Missouri Whig. "Mormon Method of Treating Cholera." May 10, 1849.

Past and Present. "Shinplasters." January 14, 2019. https://pastandpresent.com.

Peoples Tribune (Jefferson City, MO). "Death of Dr. John H. Edwards." January 5, 1876.

———. "In Memorium." February 19, 1873.

Philadelphia Branch Membership, Mormon Historic Sites, www.mormonhistoricsites.org.

Philadelphia Inquirer and National Gazette. "Died." June 4, 1849.

"Proclamation of The Twelve Apostles of The Church of Jesus Christ, of Latter Day Saints." April 6, 1845. Internet Archive. https://archive.org.

"Proclamation of the Twelve Apostles of The Church of Jesus Christ of Latter-day Saints (April 6 and October 22, 1845)." http://www.mormonhaven.com.

Read, Georgia Willis, and Ruth Gaines, eds. *Gold Rush, The Journals, Drawings, and Other Papers of J. Goldsborough Bruff April 2, 1849–July 20, 1851.* New York: Columbia University Press, 1944.

Richmond (VA) Whig and Public Advertiser. "Californians at Independence." May 29, 1849.

Ripley (OH) Bee. "The Mormons." January 31, 1852.

Saint Paul (MN) Globe. "Old Days on the Missouri." January 24, 1904.

Saturday Morning Visitor (Warsaw, MO). "Jefferson City Steam Ferry Boat." November 11, 1848.

Sayers, Edward. *Jefferson Inquirer* (Jefferson City, MO), May 19, 1849.

Smyser, H. "Dr. Smyser's Report." *Republican Banner*" (Gettysburg, PA), September 11, 1832.

Sonoma (CA) Democrat. "Sonoma District Pioneers." September 9, 1885.

State Journal (Jefferson City, MO). "The Centennial Fourth. How the Day Was Celebrated in This City." July 7, 1876.

Sunday News and Tribune (Jefferson City, MO). "History of Jefferson City Outlined for Cole County Historical Society." December 4, 1960.

Turner, William. *Voices of Missouri's Rivers.* Jefferson City: Missouri Department of Conservation, 2014.

"Utah Deaths and Burials, 1888–1946." Elizth. D. Lamb, 05 Nov 1851; citing Salt Lake City, Salt Lake, Utah, reference Pg. 4 #154; FHL microfilm 26,553. Family Search. February 10, 2018. https://familysearch.org.

Ward, Maurine Carr. "Philadelphia Pennsylvania Branch Membership: 1840–1854." *Mormon Historical Studies* 6, no. 1 (spring 2005). Salt Lake City, UH: Mormon Historic Sites Foundation. http://mormonhistoricsites.org.

Way, Frederick. *Way's Packet Directory, 1848–1983: Passenger Steamboats of the Mississippi River System Since the Advent of Photography in Mid-Continent America.* Athens: Ohio University, 1983.

Webster, Noah. *American Dictionary of the English Language*. 1828. http://webstersdictionary1828.com/Dictionary.

Weekly Herald (Madison, IN). "The Ship of Death." October 6, 1892.

Woodruff, Emma S. Collection, 1832–1919; Woodruff family miscellany; Papers of Mary Webster, 1850; Church History Library. Accessed February 21, 2019. https://catalog.churchofjesuschrist.org.

Woodruff, Wilford. Journals and papers, 1828–1898; Wilford Woodruff Journals, 1833–1898; Wilford Woodruff journal, 1847 January–1853 December; Church History Library. Accessed March 15, 2019. https://catalog.churchofjesuschrist.org.

———. Woodruff, Wilford 1807–1898. Wilford Woodruff letter, Cambridgeport, Massachusetts, to Alexander Badlam. Accessed April 15, 2019. https://catalog.churchofjesuschrist.org.

Woodstock Mercury, and Windsor County Advertiser (Woodstock, VT). "Deaths of a Family." June 1, 1849.

SURNAME INDEX

L

M

P

R

S

V

W

Y

ABOUT THE AUTHOR

A resident of Jefferson City, Missouri, Gary Elliott is a land surveyor by profession. He enjoys playing the piano, camping and hiking and researching his (or anyone's) family history. He has authored *The History of the Jefferson City and Cole County Councils of the Boy Scouts of America: 1910–1929* (Morris Publishing, 2010), and *They Came and They Went: A Brief Account of Hannibal Missouri's Early Jewish Community, and the B'nai Sholem Cemetery (Along With Those Interred There)* (Art Bookbindery Inc., 2017). He loves the challenge of separating fact from fiction. In this story, Gary has expanded his interest in history to try to unravel another historical event. He feels that "there is always a story to be told, and one does not have to be a professional writer to tell it."